Herbal Medicine

Nature's Road to Good Health and Longevity

PHILIP E. DIKA

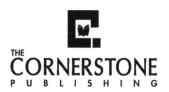

THE
CORNERSTONE
PUBLISHING

Cornerstone Publishing

A Division of Cornerstone Creativity Group LLC
Phone: +1(516) 547-4999
info@thecornerstonepublishers.com
www.thecornerstonepublishers.com

To order bulk copies of this book or to contact the author please email: dikphil_kodai@yahoo.com

DISCLAIMER

This book is not designed to undermine the usefulness of orthodox medicine. The purpose, therefore, is to provide useful information only on the subject matter hereto discussed. The author and the publishers of this book, shall not and will not be responsible for any health issues that may arise, during the course of using this book and are not liable for any condition whatsoever, either in the form of degenerate or in form of treatment, or application of the various techniques and methods of preparation. It is not the intention of the author of this book, to substitute the information therein for professional orthodox medical services, such as physician's advice, diagnosis, and treatment. Therefore, it is pertinent that you always consult your personal physician or other healthcare professionals for medical advice.

ENDORSEMENTS

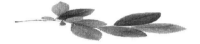

Unless we become sick or medically impaired, we do not often see any reason why good health should be taken seriously. However, in this extraordinary book, Philip has been able to prove otherwise. *Herbal Medicine: Nature's Road to Good Health and Longevity*, has unraveled the secret connection between living in good health and maintaining good health for longevity.

— RENO OMOKRI.

Herbal Medicine: Nature's Road to Good Health and Longevity, has proved a significant point to the world. The book enables us to understand the complex nature of the human body and the macromolecules in our foods. Philip has selectively put together a combination of various spices, barks, roots, leaves and herbs to formulate blends that are suitable for the natural treatment of sicknesses and diseases. This book is groundbreaking; therefore I recommend that every household should have it.

—DEBORAH CAMPBELL (RN).

FOOD FOR THOUGHT

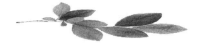

Do not be like General Naaman who said: "Are not the Abanah and the Pharpar the rivers of Damascus, better than all the waters of Israel? Could I not wash in them and be clean? So, he turned and went away in a rage" (2 Kings 5:12 NKJV).

Fortunately, for him, "his servants came near and spoke to him, and said, my father, if the prophet had told you to do something great, would you not have done it? How much more then when he says to you, wash, and be clean!" (2 Kings 5:13 NKJV)

In the end, "he went down and dipped seven times in the Jordan, according to the saying of the man of God; and his flesh was restored like the flesh of a little child, and he was clean." (2 Kings 5:14 NKJV.)

There is no harm in trial, as a trial will always convince you.

CONTENTS

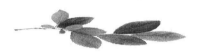

FOREWORD

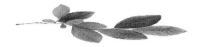

Herbal medicines are made from plants and herbs that are composed of highly specialized and organized collections of biochemical molecules, compounds and or elements with a capacity to exhibit the basic characteristics of any medicine when administered to the body, for the purpose of treatment of diseases and ailments.

In whatever form they are produced, either as solid or liquid, or a combination of both, herbal medicines are maintained as distinct entities by their mechanism of action on their various receptor organs. All herbal medicines have specific character and flavor of varying degrees. It is the combination of these that constitutes the overall potency action of the individual herbal medicine.

There are four basic properties associated with herbal medicine. These properties are in line with the nature of illness. They are cold, warm, heat and cool. The ones that are associated with warm and heat properties, are normally prescribed for cold syndrome such as aversion to cold,

cold limbs (extremities), pale tongue and slow pulse, etc. The ones associated with cool and cold properties, are prescribed for heat syndrome, such as fever, thirst, deep colored urine, red tongue, rapid pulse, etc.

Herbal medicine has been introduced here in this book, Herbal Medicine: Nature's Road to Good Health and Longevity, with an amazingly simple description of otherwise direct techniques of preparation, which have been found useful in the study of traditional native medicine on human body.

The basic concept of biochemistry and biology in this book is incredibly detailed and simple to understand. This is a valuable contribution by the author to improving the knowledge of herbal medicine. All nurses and health care professionals will find the book useful. The book is also highly recommended to every household all over the world.

Modupe Onakoya,
Registered Pharmacist.

SCRIPTURAL PERSPECTIVE

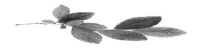

Revelation 22:2 (CEV):
> *"Then it flowed down the middle of the city's main street. On each side of the river are trees that grow a different kind of fruit each month of the year. The fruit gives life, and the leaves are used as medicine to heal the nations."*

Ezekiel 47:12 (CEV):
> *"Fruit trees will grow all along this river and produce fresh fruit every month. The leaves will never dry out, because they will always have water from the stream that flows from the temple, and they will be used for healing people."*

The above scriptures give credence and support to the powerful revelation, explanation and usefulness of the fruits, leaves, herbs and plants mentioned in this book. God, from the beginning, gave humanity the power to heal various ailments through the consumption of fruits and leaves.

As it was in the beginning, so it is presently because God remains the same yesterday today and forever. And His power and potency embedded in fruits and herbs to heal remain intact.

The author, Mr. Philip Dika, a trained biochemist with some knowledge in agricultural science and herbal medicine combined his biblical knowledge and his herbal medicine experience to put together this book as a form of manual or reference book for the usefulness of humanity.

You will find this book useful for the wealth of knowledge it contains, in the treatment, prevention and management of some common ailments, through the consumption of fruits, plants and herbs.

I strongly recommend that everyone read this powerful compendium of knowledge - for knowledge is power and knowledge is freedom.

Yemi Oyinkansola
Lead Pastor
RCCG Jesus House Antioch
CA USA.

DEDICATION

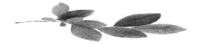

To my Lord Jesus Christ, the Author and Finisher of our faith.

To God Almighty, who freely gives wisdom to all men.

To the love of my life, my wife, Blessing M. Dika for her support, prayers and understanding throughout the course of writing this book. I love you dearly. Also, to my lovely son, David Osiozemhede Dika, for his patience, support, and encouragement. I love you dearly, my big boy.

ACKNOWLEDGMENTS

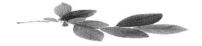

My deepest gratitude goes to God Almighty for giving me the grace, knowledge, and wisdom to write this book.

I am eternally grateful to my amazing wife, Blessing Dika and my son, David Osiozemhede Dika. Their soothing words gave me comfort and courage to continue.

More than words can truly express, I am indebted to my friends and colleagues with whom I established correspondence, which availed me many of the materials I needed for this work. I am especially grateful to Mr. Lazarus Adorolo, who assisted me in conveying my compilation of medicinal plants from Nigeria to the United States of America.

Space and time will not permit me to express my appreciation to every single person that contributed to the successful completion of this book; however, I must single out a few. Thomas Iyaogeh furnished me with some useful information. Reno Omokri encouraged me to go on with the writing of this book when I was undecided. Asifau Abigor was the force that triggered me to start writing. Mrs.

Justina Udoh and my darling wife, Blessing Dika, typed the manuscript. Words cannot express the magnitude of my gratitude to them.

I am indebted to lecturers of various departments (Biochemistry, Microbiology, Biology and Chemistry) of The Federal University of Technology, Minna, Niger State, for their tutelage. Special thanks go to lecturers at the Department of Science Laboratory Technology, Auchi Polytechnic Auchi, Nigeria, who aided in developing my neurons into physical manifestation, through impartation of knowledge.

My invaluable and immeasurable gratitude goes to my late parents, Mr. Simeon Dika and Mrs. Agatha Ayosi Dika; and to my grandparents, Mr. Yakubu Ikhioka Dika and Mr. Abba Aselimhe.

I appreciate all my siblings for their kind support: Kenneth J. O. Dika, Nelly Dika Inanemo, Christopher Dika, Julius Dika, Alexander Dika, Jane Dika Edeguare, Joy Dika Simeon, and Grace Dika Ino-Jegede. Unfortunately, Christopher and Grace walk the road no more. They are dearly missed.

Sincere gratitude to Pastor Ben Ewemie and Pastor Mrs. Becky Ewemie, Pastor Cajetan Inanila, Pastor Yemi Oyinkansola and Pastor Mrs. Comfort Oyinkansola for their prayers and support. I appreciate Pastor Yinka Somotun, Pastor Dotun Kukoyi, Pastor Kayode Fagbe Daniels, Pastor Adebayo Asogba, Pastor Ogbeide Ikhile, and all RCCG, JHA members.

Many thanks to Dr Sadiq Ikharo, President Auchi Association of America; Vice President, Constant Igiekhumhe, and every member of Auchi Association of America. I remember Engr. Joseph Inaboya, Engr. Peter Aigba, Solomon Egwaogie, my mother-in-law, Mrs. Okhuomola Aitsegame, my sister-in-law, Asifau Abigor (RN) and her husband Gabriel Abigor, Deborah Campbell (RN), Allen Bello, Asimhi S. I, Teddy & Rose Chilaka, Christiana Oiyemhonlan, Nkem Abogo-Ugwokegbe, and the rest of my friends and relatives.

INTRODUCTION

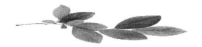

In the application of my knowledge of plant biochemistry, agricultural science and herbal medicine, I have resolved to put my pen to paper and bring together a variety of plants that are of medicinal value to man. This book is designed to educate the public, on how plants can be utilized in their natural form, to promote good health and longevity. It is also designed to meet the needs of many, who are suffering from one ailment or another, and are not responding to orthodox medicine, due to some drug resistant traits.

I have reached the conclusion that the treatment, prevention and management of many common ailments are embedded in plants. In fact, through the centuries, man has used plants to treat different kinds of sicknesses and diseases. Our ancestors drew pictures of various plants that grew around them. They knew, through observation and experience, which plants were useful or harmful to them. Their survival, in a sense, depended greatly on their knowledge of these plants. And with the passage of time, their observations and inferences paved way for the traditional study of medicinal plants, which eventually translated into modern scientific study of plants, known today, as Botany.

This knowledge of traditional herbal medicine helped our forefathers put together different spices, barks, leaves, roots, and herbs, to formulate blends that were suitable for treatment of sicknesses and diseases. This knowledge has found its way through generations in different families in the West African sub-region, Africa, and other parts of the world. My maternal grandfather was very proficient in the act of putting herbs together to formulate blends for medicinal uses, with which people were treated and cured of their ailments. It is pertinent to note that I served as my grandfather's personal assistant.

Without doubt, this book will find its usefulness in the hands of many, who will consult it for knowledge and treatment of various sicknesses and diseases, including, constipation, heart attack, migraine, obesity, diabetes, liver disease, intellectual disability, hypertension, hypotension, kidney disease, high blood pressure, hormonal imbalance, colon cancer, etc. Colon cancer, for instance, is characterized by growth from the inner wall of the large intestine due to excess fat. It is a swift, sudden killer.

Long before man was created, God knew that the devil was going to introduce sicknesses and diseases to the world; hence He decided to make plants available for man's use. That is why God said in the book of Genesis 1:11, 29, *"Let the earth bring forth grass, the herb yielding seeds, and the fruit tree yielding fruit after his kind, whose seed is in itself upon the earth; and it was so…Behold, I have given you every plant yielding seed, which is upon the face of all the earth, and every tree with seed in its fruit; you shall have them for food."*

Other Scripture references that confirm that God gave us plants for feeding and healing purposes are Ezekiel 47:12 and Revelation 22:1-2. In Ezekiel 47:12, God said, *"And on the banks on both sides of the river, there will grow all kinds of trees for food. Their leaves will not whiter nor their fruit fail, but they will bear fresh fruit every month, because the water for them flows from the sanctuary. Their fruit will be for food and their leaves for healing."* And Revelation 22:1-2 says, *"Then he showed me the river of the water of life, bright as crystal, flowing from the throne of God and of the Lamb. Through the middle of the street of the city; also on either side of the river, the tree of life with its twelve kinds of fruit, yielding its fruit each month; and the leaves of the tree were for the healing of the nations."*

Now, it is surprising how people, out of ignorance, suffer from minor ailments, like lack of energy, chronic fatigue, or acute disease conditions. In some cases, when we experience a form of tiredness, it is because of some medical issues, such as vitamin deficiency, anemia, malnutrition, high or low blood pressure, heart disease, blood circulation problems, kidney or liver diseases, digestive tract problems, constipation colitis, and diarrhea, and other focal infections, in which bacteria are localized in special organs, such as underactive thyroid gland, sinus, and the ear. When these conditions are taken care of, the body returns to a healthy state.

I have selectively put together various herbs for the prevention and treatment of sicknesses and diseases. These selections have helped my family and many others, through the ages, to survive various epidemics and plagues that have ravaged the land in time past.

During my early years, I often assisted my grandfather, who specialized in home distillation and blending of these herbal formulas as beverages, making multiple mixtures of blends, with a characteristic pleasing aroma of spicy herbs into very potent medicine for the treatment of many diseases. As a child, I was extremely interested in the practice, that I soon became skilled in the act of herbal medicine production. This I did, before I moved on impulse, to study Biochemistry.

Over the years, I have discovered that good nutrition, involving avocado and citrus fruits, which are a component of vitamin E and C respectively, can extend the life span of people who are already in their 50s. Maintaining a good health is paramount for longevity. Therefore, a daily supplement of large amount of plant based vitamin C, Vitamin E, and adequate consumption of other plant derived vitamins and minerals, with complete avoidance of sugar, and smoking, could increase the length of life and years spent in good health, by about 30 years.

This is not to say that orthodox medicine does not have its place in the treatment of sicknesses and diseases; you must at least see your doctor for diagnosis. I once read an article by Francis Ewherido, titled: *What will kill you is before you*. In the article, Ewherido noted that, on one of his visits to a former colleague and longtime friend, Assumpta Udoh, the latter told him something he found very profound because of its clarity: "Franco, by the time you are 50, the health problem that will kill you will be before you. How long you live thereafter depends on how you manage it."

Assumpta is very correct. Her grandmother was diabetic but died at the age of 98. Her 101-year-old father is asthmatic yet going strong. Last year, at the age of 100, he played exhibition tennis at the Ikoyi Club, Lagos. Ewherido went further to say that there are people whose health challenges manifest before they attain the age of 50, just as there are also people blessed with good health. You must have heard some people over 40 say, "I have not been ill in the last 20 years." Or "I have not been to the hospital for 16 years." If you are one of such, I congratulate you; however, kindly visit a hospital for checkup.

My father was never ill, except for occasional bouts of malaria. He had his first major illness at 62 and that took his life. Since 1974, my mother has been a regular at the hospital. To the glory of God, she is still kicking with all her faculties intact. She will be 85 this year. Do not assume anything when it comes to health; once you are 40 years, annual medical checkup becomes a necessity.

The checkups recommended by medical practitioners include physical examination, visual examination, blood count, urinalysis, prostate specific antigen (men above 40), chest x-ray (above 40 years), prostate scan (men above 50 years), electrocardiogram (those above 40 years), colonoscopy (men above 50 years), mammography (for women above 50 years) and some other tests.

Each of these procedures serves a particular purpose. Chest x-ray, for instance, is meant to show the state of your lungs. Chest x-rays can detect heart-related lung conditions, cancer, infections like tuberculosis and pneumonia, or air collecting in the space around a lung, among others.

Blood sugar level is for all persons 40 years and above, especially people from families where there is a history of diabetes. In fact, such a person should have been doing their checkup long before age 40. Normal blood sugar level is between 70 and 99 fasting (that is, when you wake up in the morning) and not more than 140 two hours after meal at all times. Early detection of high blood sugar can help you ward off diabetes and its attendant complications. Thankfully, blood sugar test is one of those tests you can do at home with your test kits.

Like blood sugar, blood pressure can also be easily checked at home with the test kits. Normal blood pressure is diastolic 80 and systolic 120. Once your systolic is 130 and above, you have high blood pressure. Of course, as people grow older, these figures can be higher and still be okay. But you must consult your doctor if you have high blood pressure.

Some people develop migraines when their blood pressure

rises. The consequences of blood pressure are mostly devastating. It can lead to stroke, which results in partial or total paralysis and, possibly, death. People with high blood pressure should check their blood pressure regularly and take their blood pressure medication regularly. It is a silent killer.

Once you attain the age of 40, you must, of necessity, adjust your lifestyle to stay healthy. This includes the quality and quantity of food you consume. In your younger days, your metabolism was higher, and you could burn off carbohydrates (sugar) easily. This however changes as you grow older; so, you need to cut down on the quantity of food you consume per time, to reduce the work of your aging internal organs. The common saying, "Eat like a king in the morning, a prince in the afternoon and a pauper in the evening" might not apply to some people in their 50s or older. They should simply obey their bodies and eat little when it is necessary.

Let me state unequivocally that you also must be wary of the common saying that "you can never be wrong with fruits." Unless you understand your body very well, you can go horribly wrong with fruits. People with diabetic tendencies cannot consume "sweet" fruits like banana, oranges, pineapple, etc., in large quantities. They will either consume these fruits in strict moderation or totally abstain from eating them. You also need to know what goes well with your body. For instance, some people are allergic to certain fruits.

Finally, in your younger days, sports and exercise might have been simply for fun and recreation. Once you hit 40, however, exercising becomes a matter of life and death. For many people, it is no longer fun, because of aching joints and aging internal organs; but you must exercise or perish slowly. You should understand that the whole essence of exercise at this age is to stay healthy, give a reasonably good account of yourself sexually (for men) and shed some weight, if possible.

For men over 40, building muscles should not be the motivation for exercising. Who are you trying to impress? Certainly not your wife of 20 years or more, who is more interested in your "financial muscles" that can give her financial security over time. This is also connected to why people above 40 years are advised to walk briskly (not jog) about 30 minutes every day.

Beyond your physician, let your personal doctor (your body) be your guide, so you do not slump and die prematurely. If you go to any sporting facility, you will see some sexagenarians and septuagenarians jogging, while people in their 30s are walking. It is partly because of the instructions from their bodies. Some of those old men jogging have been doing it religiously for over 40 years.

Listen to your body, but exercise you must, as Ewherido's cousin, Dr. (Mrs.) Martina would always say, "It's good to exercise regularly because, if the benefits of exercising were put in a pill, it would be the best selling pill worldwide." Ewherido continued by saying that many young people in their 40s and 50s are dropping dead with alarming rapidity. Please, do not swell the number because of your carelessness or negligence. *Mutatis mutandis*, which is to say, what is true and correct in one part of the world is also true and correct in other parts. If it happens in Nigeria, it can also be said in America or elsewhere.

CHAPTER ONE

THE COMPLEX NATURE OF THE HUMAN BODY

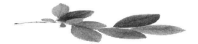

The human body is made up of cells, tissues, and organs. Like cells are grouped together to form tissues, just as two or more different tissues may align to form an organ. Examples of such tissues are the muscular, the epithelial, the connective, the skeletal, and the nervous tissues. Muscular, nervous, fatty (adipose), skeletal, epidermal, and connective tissues, for instance, come together to form the hands and the legs, which are organs themselves, while the epithelial, muscular, connective, and other types of tissues, form the different organs in the alimentary canal.

The mouth, gullet, stomach, intestines, liver, and pancreas are organs associated with feeding and the digestion of food. All these organs work together to form the digestive system.

There is a collection of sub-integrated systems in the human body. These include the circulatory, the nervous, the locomotive, the excretory, and the respiratory systems.

All these systems must work together in a concerted effort to form a unified system, known as the human being. This explains why, in Biochemistry, there is a subject that deals with the metabolism of individual substances, such as carbohydrates, amino acids and fatty acids in the body on the one hand; and on the other hand, a subject that deals collectively with the metabolism of all the substances in the body, called integrated metabolism or intermediary metabolism and regulation. This is where we talk about the path of dietary compounds after digestion and absorption, and the manner in which these compounds are channeled into other products.

This subject encompasses a wide range, that seeks to address the metabolic pathways taken by molecules of complex structures and attempts to facilitate an understanding of the interrelationship and mechanism that regulates the flow of metabolites through the different pathways. In common parlance, metabolic pathways fall into three categories. The first is the anabolic pathway, which gives rise to the synthesis of compounds constituting the body structure and machinery, such as proteins, carbohydrates, and fats. In this process, consumption of energy, which the pathway itself cannot provide, is required. The second category is the catabolic pathway. This is the oxidative process that generates free energy in form of high energy phosphate bond compound or reducing equivalent in the oxidative phosphorylation process associated with respiratory chain.

Previously, metabolism pathways were simply divided

into two categories: anabolism and catabolism. Deeper understanding of the biochemistry of metabolism pathways, however, has opened us up to the existence of a third pathway – the amphibolic pathway. This amphibolic pathway has different functions and they occur at critical control points, known as crossroads of metabolism, where they act as linkage between anabolic and catabolic pathways. An example of this is the Citric Acid Cycle (CAC). The biomedical significance of this is that a good knowledge of metabolism in the normal human system is a prerequisite for proper understanding of abnormal metabolism, with respect to many diseases.

Normal and Abnormal Metabolism

The existence of abnormal metabolism implies that there is normal metabolism. What therefore is normal and abnormal metabolism? Normal metabolism includes the variation and adaption in metabolic processes, due to periods of starvation, exercise, pregnancy, and lactation. Whereas abnormal metabolism results from a number of dysfunctions in the human system, such as nutritional deficiency or abnormal secretion of hormones, arising from genetic deficiencies, such as diabetes mellitus and metabolic deficiencies associated with inability to effectively metabolize glucose, as a result of either lack of insulin or biochemically defective insulin.

The point here is that one body part cannot function properly without the proper functioning of other parts.

The body system is a group of different parts that work together to achieve a common purpose. For example, the cardiovascular system works to circulate blood through the body, while the respiratory system gives oxygen to the body. These body systems are interconnected and dependent on one another to function effectively. The brain and the nervous system coordinate to give signals to the heart to enable it beat. Also, the skeletal system utilizes the nutrients it acquires from the digestive system to develop strong and healthy bones and these are concerted efforts.

It is therefore pertinent that adequate care is taken to ensure the body is given proper attention by way of eating the right food and taking the right medicine to keep the body in good health and prevent sicknesses and diseases.

We will now consider vital organs of the human body and how they function.

Organs of the Body

The Skin

The skin has three layers. The **epidermis**, which is the outermost layer, provides a waterproof barrier and creates our skin tone. The **dermis** is located beneath the epidermis, and contains tough connective tissues, hair follicles, and sweat glands. The **deeper subcutaneous tissue** (hypodermis) is made up of fat and connective tissues.

The skin color is created by special cells called melanocytes, which are located in the epidermis. These melanocytes produce the pigment called, melanin, which prevents the penetration of the ultra-violet rays of sunlight. Also present in the epidermis is keratin, a protein which is responsible for the toughness and flexibility of the skin.

The human skin is very important in that, it helps humans to maintain a constant body temperature; hence they are regarded as homoeothermic. They have a constant body temperature of 37^0C or 98^0F. Heat is produced in the body by tissue respiration, the activities of the internal organs and muscular exercise. This heat is transported to all parts of the body through blood circulation, and the body is kept warm. When there is excessive heat in the system, it is normally expelled through urination, defecation, exhalation, conduction, convection, radiation and sweating.

In humans, the highest temperature possible before death occurs is 42^0C or 107.6^0F, and the lowest temperature is 27^0C or 70^0F. This narrow temperature range is critical as it affects the efficiency of our body's metabolic functions. It can, however, deviate significantly from one value to another, depending on whether we are resting, exercising, or partaking in other physical activities.

These activities cause a small variation in our body temperature, which our heat regulating mechanism efficiently copes with. But in disease conditions, the body temperature is elevated beyond the normal range, causing the heat and cooling system of the body to break down.

When the body is attacked by malaria, for instance, there is a recurrent cycle of chill, fever, and profuse sweating. It occurs in a 48 or 72-hour cycle, depending on the species of the plasmodium parasite involved. Fever is caused by toxins released into the blood by the malaria parasite. These toxins have a direct effect on the hypothalamus. Heat-producing mechanisms, like vasoconstriction and hair erection, become active and produce a lot of heat.

Although the temperature of the internal body is raised, the skin remains cold. This condition is known as a chill and the patients usually shake violently. When the body temperature reaches its height, the patient starts to feel hot. This is the crisis period. If the temperature remains unattended to, the patient usually dies of dehydration. But, if the fever breaks, the sweating period falls sharply, with profuse sweating, and he or she begins to feel normal again. Unless treated with the required herbs, the entire process will restart in a cyclic pattern which may lead to death. Temperature is a physical quantity, which characterizes the thermal state of a body. That is why the thermometer is used to check the body's temperature to determine the wellness level.

The Kidneys

There are two bean-shaped kidneys in the human body. They are irregularly situated on the upper wall of the stomach, the right kidney being more noticeable than the left. They are held in position by a mass of fatty tissues. Lying above each kidney is a conical adrenal gland, which is an endocrine gland (gland that produces secretions). These glands consist of a peripheral cortex and a middle medulla.

The medulla is responsible for adrenalin production, as the cortex is responsible for the production of a collection of hormones, which are together known as corticosterones. It is also responsible for producing little amounts of hormones that control the development of secondary sexual characteristics.

In an unexpected, and often dangerous situation, requiring immediate action, or fear, danger and emergency, adrenalin is released into the blood, which activates the activities of the sympathetic nervous system, and many other organs, thereby increasing muscular activity and the rate of heartbeat, as well as increased sugar level of the blood.

Adrenalin prepares the body to respond to these unexpected situations. This affects the pupils of the eyes, as they become dilated, and the visceral muscles. Hence adrenalin is known as an emergency hormone or a shock absorber.

The kidneys function to remove unwanted nitrogenous substances, like urea and ammonia, as well as dissolved carbon dioxide, from the bloodstream. They also get rid of excess water and salt and keep the osmotic concentration of the blood constant. In addition to these, they play a role in the regulation of blood pressure, producing red blood cells and filtering waste products from the body. In this process, blood first passes through the tiny blood vessels in the cortex, which remove waste products from the blood. The filtered blood flows into small tubes (in the medulla) that reabsorb the nutrient and water that the body needs. The filtered and replenished blood returns to the circulation, and the left-over waste or by product (urine) is collected in the renal pelvis. Urine drains through the urethra into the bladder, where it is stored until it is expelled from the body.

The kidney is susceptible to a wide range of disorders. However, since one kidney is adequate for good health, the disorder is seldom life-threatening, unless it affects both kidneys. Such disorders associated with the kidneys include congenital abnormality, such as horseshoe kidney (usually common and harmless). Serious, inherited kidney disorders include polycystic disease, in which the cysts enlarge until the whole kidney is destroyed. It is common amongst middle aged people, producing abnormal sweating, pains, and blood in the urine, known as hematuria. As the disease progresses, hypertension, and kidney failure set in. There is no effective treatment for this, other than kidney transplant or dialysis.

Other medical conditions associated with the kidneys are kidney cyst and blood vessel damage, caused by shock or hemolytic urine syndrome (urine in the blood). Diabetes mellitus can also cause kidney disorder. Glomerulonephritis, as well as allergic reaction due to medication or long-term treatment with analgesic and antibiotic, can destroy the kidney.

Moreover, metabolic disorders, like hyperuricemia (high level of urea in the blood) may cause kidney stone, leading to gout. In this condition, uric acid crystal is deposited in the joints. This also can be caused by an inborn error of metabolism. Hyperuricemia can also be caused by leukemia (cancer of the blood) or medication that induces the kidney to produce uric acid, e.g. diuretic drugs. It can also be caused by large amount of purine in the diet (that is, too much consumption of organ meat like liver and kidney).

Hypertension can also result in kidney damage. Other causes are kidney tumor, kidney cancer, kidney failure. Kidney stone, also known as calculus, is a little hard crystalline mass formed in the body cavity from certain substances in the fluid such as the bile, saliva and even in the urine. This stone can occur in the gall bladder and bile duct. Most of the kidney stones are made up of calcium oxalate or other crystalline salt formation of these stones and can be associated with oxalic acid found in leafy vegetables and coffee, or high level of calcium in the blood from hyperthyroidism or chronic dehydration.

In the abdomen, there is a location called the pyloric region, where the stomach is connected to or opens into the small intestine (duodenum) by means of a U-shaped loop. Between the arms of the U-shaped loop, lies the pancreas, and scattered in the pancreatic cells, are a group of granular cells, known as the islet of Langerhans that secretes the hormone insulin, which regulates the glucose level in the blood. When there is a deficiency of this hormone (insulin), diabetes is inevitable. This is a disease condition caused by too much sugar or glucose in the blood.

There are many types of diabetes. Two of them are type 1 and type 2 diabetes. Type 1 diabetes occurs when the body's immune system attacks and causes destruction of the beta cells that produce insulin in the pancreas (islets of Langerhans). This results in insufficient or no production of insulin to regulate the sugar or glucose level in the blood, leading to accumulation of glucose in the blood (diabetes mellitus). Type 1 diabetes manifests in sudden weight loss, incessant urination, tiredness, blurry vision, insatiable hunger, and lack of strength.

Type 2 diabetes occurs when there is inability of the body to utilize or produce enough insulin. In this case, the insulin produced is not enough to efficiently transport glucose into the cells for use as energy generation. The body becomes resistant to insulin and glucose, and starts building up in the system, which consequently leads to the excretion of glucose or sugar in the urine.

Fortunately, in modern times, patients suffering from diabetes can now lead a normal life by taking proper diet that is incorporated with Gynura procumbens (longevity spinach or longevity greens). This is a herb/vegetable that contains special properties, which have the ability to improve health and fix conditions, such as high cholesterol levels, diabetes and high blood pressure.

The Liver

The liver helps in the digestion of food, as well as removal of waste products from the body. When there is excess of protein in the diet, it is necessary to get rid of it. This is because there is no organ or tissue in the body where the excess can be stored.

Surplus amino acids produced due to high protein diet are transported to the liver. Here, each amino acid is broken down into amino group ($-NH2$) and a carbon group, known as keto acid. The amino group is converted to ammonia, which is harmful to the body cells, but it is very soon converted again to harmless urea. The keto acid is converted to glycogen (carbohydrate) or fat which can be used by the body on a later day. This whole process of breakdown of amino acid is known as deamination. The urea, which is produced, is removed afterwards by the kidneys.

In addition to the process described above, the liver is equally responsible for the conversion of foreign substances, which may have entered the body via ingestion or other means, to harmless or inactive forms that can be easily excreted.

Some of these foreign substances are drugs ingested through the mouth or through injection, preservatives, industrial chemicals used in laboratories and water treatment, and of course, pollution. Examples of such chemicals are silica dust, particles of asbestos, carbon monoxide, hydrogen sulfide and ammonia. Others are produced by bacterial action on food retained for a long time in the large intestine. 90% of these substances are toxic and could damage the cells.

The liver also carries out a process known as detoxification. That is when these toxic substances are converted to nonpoisonous or inactive forms, which are consequently excreted by the kidneys in the urine. However, some of them are retained in the liver and secreted into the intestine in the bile, before they are finally excreted as feces.

However, in disease conditions, such as Hepatitis C, liver cancer, liver cirrhosis, the functionality of the liver becomes impaired and, if not treated, can lead to liver failure. The following are symptoms of liver failure: muscle loss, itching, bleeding, or bruising easily, vomiting blood, passing black stool, forgetfulness, confusion, nausea, loss of appetite, extreme fatigue, weakness, jaundice and bleeding in the stomach.

The Heart

The heart is considered the most powerful of all the organs in the circulatory system. It carries out its function incessantly, like a muscular pump, and keeps the blood in continuous circulation. Each pumping action of the heart is termed a heartbeat. Averagely, when at rest, man has about 72 heartbeats per minute. This can increase to about 100 and above during activity or excitement. The heartbeat can be counted by feeling the pulse at the wrist. When the heart beats 72 times in a minute, it follows that, in an hour, it beats 4,320 times. In 24 hours, it beats 103,680 times; and accordingly, 37,843,200 times in one year. At the age of 90, the average individual would have had about 3.4 billion heartbeats!

In carrying out its function of constantly pumping blood throughout the body, the heart always utilizes energy. The heart gives excellent ceaseless services for a long period of time without stopping. It works every moment of everyday, as long as life lasts, and only rests within a fraction of seconds between beats. Should our heart stop for more than a few seconds, we would automatically lose consciousness, and go into coma. And if it does not get started within a few seconds or minutes, it will lead to irreversible brain damage and, eventually, death.

Sadly, however, this vital organ of the human body, which keeps our blood in constant circulation, can be weakened by various diseases and different forms of abuse.

From the beginning (embryonically) the heart is modified into blood vessels, which in the act of looping, are transformed into a complex four-chambered organ from a straight tube-like structure. This four-chambered organ is divided into two upper chambers, the auricles and two lower chambers, the ventricles. These four are together known as the left auricles and the left ventricles, and right auricles and right ventricles. They continuously work together in complete harmony, pumping an average of about 6 liters of blood in the entire body; and this whole volume passes through the heart, once in every 100 beats.

Man is said to display a complete double circulation. This implies that for one complete circulation to happen, blood must pass through the heart twice; each time, going through a separate pathway. These pathways are two and are referred to as the pulmonary circulation and the systemic circulation. The pulmonary circulation is between the heart and the lungs, while the systemic circulation is between the heart and every other part of the body.

In one complete circulation, blood from one part of the body enters the heart for the first time, and then sent to the lungs for oxygenation; after which it is brought back to the heart for the second time for onward distribution to all parts of the body. This is the sequence involved in double circulation and it is a closed circulation system, in that, there is no mixing up of the oxygenated blood and deoxygenated blood in the heart. Oxygenated blood is confined to the left side of the heart, while deoxygenated blood is confined to the right side of the heart.

Also, the heart has its own special circulation to supply blood to its muscle tissues – these are the coronary arteries. The most common cardiovascular problem in man is the coronary artery disease. It is characterized by a buildup of cholesterol-filled plaque in the coronary arteries. In this condition, over the cause of many years, the arteries get blocked by fatty acid, in the same way water pipes get blocked with calcium deposits when hard water passes through it. It is a process, which often starts slowly in childhood so that, by age 20, there is gradual accumulation of fatty streaks which may be visible in the arteries.

By age 40, the arteries may be halfway blocked. In most cases, there are no symptoms at all, until it reaches an advanced stage of about 70% blockage at age 60. At this point, the blood vessels in the coronary arteries become narrow. This leads to a corresponding reduction in the supply of blood to the muscles in the heart, which then reduces the flow of oxygen and nutrients to the heart. In the passage of time, as fatty deposits continue to block the artery, the muscles that were hitherto supplied by the blood vessels die, leading to coronary artery disease. Coronary artery disease can lead to heart attack, stroke, or even death.

The heart muscle that is short of oxygen causes chest pain, pressure, or a certain kind of discomfort, called angina pectoris. The heart needs a lot of oxygen during excitement, exercise, and stress or when eating a heavy meal. In coronary artery disease, narrow blood vessels keep the extra blood with oxygen from getting to the heart due to blockage. This condition is called arteriosclerosis. Research has shown that a high fiber dietary intake lowers the risk of coronary heart attack. Cereal fiber is particularly beneficial for this condition.

When blood pressure is maintained at 140/90 or higher, a person is said to be hypertensive or suffer from high blood pressure. It may be caused by hardening and narrowing of the blood vessels. It can also result from kidney disease, tumors of the adrenal gland, and pregnancy; and can develop in a person of any age. Signs of coronary artery blockage include high blood pressure, pain in the heart region, and physical exhaustion after an exercise involving climbing of the stairs, or a steep mountain. Heart palpitation is also one of the signs.

When the heart beats, and there is a contraction of the auricles, a high pressure is created in the blood vessels inside the auricles, resulting in the folding of the bicuspid and tricuspid valves, with the valves pointing downward and backward to the ventricles and allowing blood flow into the ventricles from the auricles. This is the diastolic process. In the systolic process, the two ventricles contract, giving rise to the pushing of blood into the two trunks of the main arteries of the heart and subsequently letting the blood out of the heart. It is this diastolic and systolic process that enables the blood pressure to be established.

Symptoms of atherosclerosis are dizziness, defect in memory, buzzing sound in the ears, prickling hands, pain in the thoracic region (chest), cramp, especially in the calf and cold in the extremities.

The Lungs

The lungs are the organs where respiration (exchange of gases) takes place. Oxygen, being part of the air, we breathe, is required for the lungs to perform their functions. Hence, the lungs are known as the respiratory organs since they allow oxygen flow into the blood and simultaneously give out carbon dioxide. Even though the structure of the lungs is complicated, they have been designed by God, to efficiently carry out their functions.

During respiration, two notable events occur - inhalation and exhalation. Through inhalation, which is breathing in, air is drawn from the atmosphere into the lungs via the nostrils. While in exhalation, which is breathing out, air in the lungs, which has been utilized, is expelled via the nostrils, accompanied by some water vapor.

The oxygen contained in the inhaled air, by means of diffusion goes into the bloodstream in the capillaries around the alveoli. This occurs when oxygen concentration of the blood is much lower than that of the air in the alveoli. Therefore, the oxygen binds with the hemoglobin to form what is known as oxyhemoglobin or oxygenated blood. While that in which the oxygen is depleted, is known as deoxygenated blood. For this process to continue, oxyhemoglobin must be reconverted to hemoglobin to make provision for the binding of oxygen.

The carbon dioxide that is formed because of metabolic activities in the cells diffuses into the blood. This carbon dioxide is transported in the bloodstream as bicarbonate ions. When the bicarbonate ions get to the lungs, they decompose to give rise to carbon dioxide, which eventually diffuses into the air sacs, since the concentration of carbon dioxide in the air sacs is lower than that in the blood. By the action of the diaphragm, intercostal muscles, sternum and the thoracic cavity, the lungs are forced to contract, leading to an increase in the pressure of the air in the lungs and the air or carbon dioxide is thus released via the respiratory passages.

Hemoglobin is the oxygen-carrying pigment in the red blood cell. It is a protein that is made up of four subunits. Each of these subunits has one molecule of heme. Heme is an iron-containing porphyrin derivative. The polypeptide is collectively called globin. This implies that globin is obtained from the polypeptide chain. When put together, we have hemoglobin. In normal hemoglobin, everything works perfectly well. But during abnormal situations, such as defect in the genetic makeup that controls the expression of hemoglobin, certain disorders do occur. These disorders are many but I will restrict myself to discuss the most common – sickle cell anemia.

Originally, hemoglobin is characterized into the alpha and the beta chains. The alpha chain contains 141 amino acid residues, and the beta chain contains 146 amino acid residues, with a molecule of heme attached to each chain. The molecule of heme hangs between two of histidine residues and its iron atom is causally linked to one of the histidine residues. The other histidine residues are also associated with the iron atom, but with a space between them, where the oxygen molecules appear to be connected into the chain to bind with the hemoglobin for oxygenation.

In cases of hemoglobinopathies (genetic defects of the hemoglobin), sickle cell anemia has been implicated as the most common variant. In sickle cell anemia, the alpha (&) polypeptide chains are normal but the beta (B) polypeptide chains are abnormal, because there is a replacement of one glutamic acid residue by a valine residue at position 6 of the 146 amino acid chain sequences coding for the beta polypeptide chain. This disease is predominant in certain parts of the world. For example, in West Africa, it is found in as many as 25 percent of the population, thereby further reducing the life expectancy of such individuals.

Problems associated with this disease normally starts from age 5-6 months, and a series of health issues like pain, swelling in the extremities, stroke, and bacterial infections, may manifest. And as the patient gets older, severe long-term pain may set in. Life expectancy for people with sickle cell anemia is between 40-60 years, depending on which part of the world they find themselves. Management of this disease may include infection control or prevention, with adequate consistent vaccination and antibiotics, high intake of fluid, pain killer and a good folate supplementation. Folate is the natural form of vitamin B9 (Pteroylmonoglutamic acid). Another form of vitamin B9 is folic acid, which is synthetically produced.

From the beginning, folic acid was thought to be better absorbed than the natural folate. However, a supplement containing a variety of folate rich foods has been proven to be amazingly effective. When folic acid is taken, majority of it is not converted to the active form of vitamin B9, in the digestive system. Instead, it is converted in the liver or other tissues. In summary, high levels of un-metabolized folic acid may have a negative effect on the health of an individual by increasing the risk of cancer or hiding the deficiency of vitamin B12, which may become a pathological condition.

When hemoglobin is exposed to carbon monoxide, a reaction occurs, resulting in the formation of carboxyhemoglobin. This is because the affinity of oxygen for hemoglobin is much less than the affinity of carbon monoxide for hemoglobin. Consequently, carbon-monoxide displaces oxygen in binding with hemoglobin, thereby reducing the oxygen carrying capacity of the hemoglobin. So, instead of oxygen being transported in the bloodstream, carbon-monoxide is transported, resulting in irreversible brain damage, unconsciousness, and even death.

Since carbon-monoxide is colorless, odorless, and tasteless, people can be easily overcome by it without any warning. Many people have died in their car garages, while running their car engines with the garage door closed or when there is a fire outbreak resulting in heavy pollution, due to incomplete combustion of carbon.

Oxygen is the most important element that we need to survive; therefore, it is extremely dangerous to be deprived of it even for about 10-15 minutes. Reduced oxygen in the brain occurs when there is drowning, choking, suffocating, cardiac arrest, brain injury, stroke, and carbon-monoxide as aforementioned.

The brain is one of the most active organs of the body, even though it accounts for a ridiculously small portion of our body weight. It is divided into three main parts, which are the fore brain, the mid brain, and the hind brain. The fore brain consists of the cerebrum which is the largest part of the brain. It is made up of the right and left cerebral hemispheres that are separated by a deep furrow, called the median fissure, which is connected by a band of fibers, the corpus callosum. The cerebrum is associated with higher brain function, such as the ability to learn and exhibit intelligent behavior, like making good and correct responses. It is also the center of memory, will-power, reasoning, judgment, and imagination.

It is common knowledge that our bodies need some care to be healthy and grow well. To achieve this, we need good food and exercise. The same applies to the brain. To keep the brain in good condition, we need to maintain a balance of the elements that can affect the brain function and recovery if there is a deficiency. This is important because blood carries oxygen to the brain and oxygen is vital for brain growth and healing.

To maintain proper brain function, therefore, a critical balance of oxygen, carbon-dioxide and nitric acid levels is required for circulation. This is why when we visit hospitals, nurses often clip a certain piece of device on our finger to read the oxygen level. This device is called pulse oximeter. It gives an overview of how much oxygen is in our bloodstream. Because of its importance, this pulse oximeter reading is now regarded as the fifth vital sign, in addition to the regular four vital signs of temperature, blood pressure, heart rate and breathing rate.

Shortage or deficiency of oxygen in the brain is rarely noticeable but can however result in poor brain function and accelerated risk of dementia. Other risk factors are hypotension or hypertension, high cholesterol, diabetes, heart disease, smoking and alcoholism. In most cases, even when you think you are breathing normally, the brain may not be getting enough oxygen, because it utilizes a whole lot of oxygen to carry out its function and it is very sensitive to any slight decrease in the oxygen level, and will not perform optimally when oxygen level is low. Essentially, the brain consists of cells called the neurons.

CHAPTER TWO

THE MECHANISM OF ACTION OF MACROMOLECULES IN FOODS

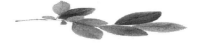

The main purpose of eating food is to generate energy, stay alive and be in good health. The macromolecules we have in our foods are proteins, nucleic acid (DNA), carbohydrates and lipids (fats and oils). The protease enzymes act on proteins to give amino acid. Amylases act on carbohydrates to give glucose, with the action of ptyalin, which acts on cooked starches to break them down to more complex sugars in the presence of a neutral or alkaline medium, which is provided by the saliva in the mouth. Lipases, on the other hand, act on lipids to give fatty acid and glycerol.

Esterification of nucleosides will produce nucleic acid by the joining of the nucleotide's pentose. Further action on glucose by the dehydrogenase enzyme will produce pyruvate and pyruvate dehydrogenase enzyme will act on pyruvate to produce acetyl CoA for energy generation. The calorific value of carbohydrate is ½ less than that of fat and may defer considerably in the proportions of its diets. On the average, western diet may comprise 200gm of carbohydrate, 80 gm of protein, 70 gm of fat and the basal usage of calories is about 1700 calories a day.

An average man, who is physically active, requires a daily intake of about 5000 calories. Excess calories, whether in the form of protein, fat, or carbohydrate, are converted to lipid and stored in the liver and muscles as glycogen, ready to be mobilized during starvation, fasting and shortage of food.

To be in good health and vitality, therefore, nature requires us to maintain a particularly good digestive system. The digestive system consists of the mouth, esophagus, liver, gallbladder, bile duct, pancreatic duct, pancreas, and the colon - which is divided into ascending, transverse and descending colon. The descending colon is linked to the rectum, which opens to the outside. In the event that one of these parts of the digestive system has a problem, the whole body begins to degenerate.

The Digestive Process

After eating, food stays in the stomach for about four hours before digestion is complete. But when food fails to digest, and waste is not eliminated within a given time, the food becomes poison in the stomach, which then begins to develop into disease conditions, such as constipation, kidney disease, liver disease, insomnia, low IQ, heart attack, eye disease, pile, diabetes, hypertension, colon cancer, obesity, migraine, headache, hormonal imbalance, rheumatism, asthma, appendicitis, arthritis, cancer, prostatitis and so on.

The stimuli that first trigger the digestive system are the aroma and sight of food; and just by having a taste of the food, ptyalin, an amylase enzyme secreted in the mouth, is set in motion to start the break down process of the food. As earlier stated, the digestive process in the stomach lasts for about four hours per meal, depending on the type and quantity of food consumed. The gastric juice, which is produced by the gastric glands in the stomach, also facilitates digestion. This gastric juice has two important enzymes known as pepsin and rennin, which require an acid medium, such as hydrochloric acid to work in. This acid stops the action of ptyalin that has been going on in the gullet and at the same time helps to sterilize the stomach by killing the putrefying bacteria in the stomach.

The enzyme, pepsin, a protease, causes the breakdown of proteins into protease and peptones that are intermediate products in the digestion of proteins. It is this pepsin that causes the coagulation of milk into thin curds, known as caseinogen (soluble milk protein) and subsequently converting it into casein (insoluble milk protein). The cells that produce enzymes in the walls of the small intestine also produce an alkaline liquid called intestinal juice, which contains enzymes that act on the remaining food in the alimentary canal to complete the process of digestion, by converting the complex sugars to glucose. This is the end of digestion of carbohydrates.

Similarly, the enzyme protease (erepsin) causes the reduction of peptones and polypeptides to amino acids, which are also the end products of protein digestion. The acetyl CoA, as aforementioned, is also an important constituent of the intestinal juice that participates in the metabolism of carbohydrate lipids and protein, whose function is to deliver the acetyl group to the citric acid cycle for energy generation, via the oxidative process. Glucose, amino acid and fatty acid are collected in the small intestine and then entered into the bloodstream via blood vessels called villi through a process of absorption.

Obesity Indicators

Over-consumption of carbohydrate foods has been identified as the common cause of obesity and associated nutritional disorders. Other factors that contribute to obesity are lack of exercise, environmental conditions, genetic defects or epigenetic health status, poor sleep, emotional state, stress, and medication. When the body mass index (BMI) is 30 or more, the person is said to be obese. A healthy BMI is considered to be between 18.5 and 24.9. When the BMI is less than 18.5, a person is considered underweight; but when a person's BMI is between 25 and 29.9, then they are considered overweight.

The risk of obesity is higher in men with waist larger than

40 inches and in women with waist larger than 35 inches. Body Mass Index (BMI) is a calculation that indicates the healthiness of an individual's weight. This reveals the amount of fat a person carries, using the person's height and weight. For instance, if your height is 70 inches and your weight is 206 lbs., you can use the following formulae to determine your BMI:

BMI Calculation:

IMPERIAL SYSTEM.	METRIC SYSTEM
$$\dfrac{703 \times \text{wt in (lbs)}}{(\text{ht in inches})^2}$$	$$\dfrac{\text{wt (kg)}}{\text{ht (m}^2)}$$
$$\dfrac{703 \times 206 \text{ lbs}}{70^2}$$	EX. W = 94kg; H = 176 cm $$176\text{cm}/100 = 1.76\text{m}$$ BMI $\dfrac{94\text{kg}}{1.76^2} = 30$
BMI = 29.6	**BMI = 30**

Metric System: Weight in kg and height in meters

The simplest way to calculate your BMI is to first measure your height in centimeter and convert it to meter by dividing the value by 100. This is because 100 cm= 1m. Example, if your height is 176 cm, then in meters, it is 1.76m. To convert pounds (lbs.) to kilograms (kg) divide by 2.2

To convert kilograms (kg) to pounds (lbs.) multiply by 2.2

To convert meters to centimeters, you multiply by 100.

Obesity, from a genetic point of view, occurs when changes in gene expression happens without any modification to the DNA sequence of the amino acid polypeptide chain. Examples of such changes are epigenetic changes associated with obesity that has to do with exposure to chemicals that are disruptive to the endocrine system, thereby resulting in the malfunctioning of the endocrine system, causing over-secretion or under-secretion of hormones. These exposures occur early in life and activate changes in the physiological process, which can linger till old age. Individual factors also include knowing what to and what not to eat, attitude to life and behavioral pattern. Other factors like schools and workplace food options and opportunity for physical activities, as well as accessing health promotion services like hospitals, clinics, gym, and wellness programs, are also considered.

Importance of Fiber-rich Foods

In the alimentary canal of man, the caecum is absent. This means that humans cannot digest cellulose. However, it is pertinent that we include plant produce in our food or diet, as this will give bulk to the food and facilitate its passage through the alimentary canal. Foods that serve this purpose are known as roughages.

Roughages are fiber-rich foods and are required for easy digestion of food ingested and easy egestion of solid waste from the body to avoid poisoning the whole body. People who eat *eba* (cassava pudding) , unfiltered *garri,* tapioca (made from cassava or yucca root), whole grains, fruits, vegetables, bean nuts, seeds, other forms of roughages etc., and take large quantity of water regularly, maintain an incredibly good digestive system. With the help of fiber-rich foods, the body can get rid of waste products faster and prevent re-absorption of toxic substances (which can cause cancer, tumor growth and other terrible diseases) in the body. We must, therefore, be careful and intentional about what we eat.

In facilitating the passage of the food through the intestine after eating, fiber prevents the concentration of localized pressures and therefore reduces the average gastric residence time (which is the interval between when food is eaten and when it is passed out as waste). Gastric residence time for the occidental is about 72 hours whereas that of an African is about 48 hours. Therefore, the shorter the residence time, the less possibility of attack by gut or gastric microorganism, thereby reducing flatulence. Fiber affects the secretion of bile, which tends to reduce blood cholesterol levels. Adequate fiber in the diet helps prevent diverticulitis of the colon.

Crude fiber is an organic component of the food we eat, and it is composed of cellulose, hemicellulose, plant gum, mucilage, and small amount of lignin. These are altogether known as roughage. It is in the portion of plant food that cannot be completely digested by the human digestive system, because humans lack the caecum, which harbors the bacteria that produces the enzyme cellulases, that is responsible for the digestion of cellulose.

Caution with Food Combinations

Dr. (Mrs.) Lopsam, a naturopath/acupuncturist (LINM, LNHC), in her article titled, *Wrong Food Combination*, said that the source of many diseases and the reason why diseases persist is because of wrong food combinations. She added that to live long and enjoy good health, one should study proper food combination, because, according to her, when food is properly combined, the whole body enjoys. If, however, food is wrongly combined, certain abnormalities arise, the liver suffers so much and, in some cases, it gives up, leading to severe illnesses or even death, in worst cases.

Dr. Lopsam went further to say that, for example, millions of people enjoy beans and fried ripe plantain, and that, as a matter of fact, beans and ripe plantain is so delicious, such that hardly does anyone resist it. She added however that it is one of the most wrongly combined foods. She said cooking or combining foods like beans with unripe plantain has no problems. In fact, it is a perfect combination, which makes digestion easy. However, the same plantain, when it is ripe, becomes fruit. Check the difference.

1. Unripe plantain is not sweet
2. You cannot eat it raw
3. Ripe plantain is overly sweet
4. You can eat it raw.

This explains that cooking ripe plantain on fire turns the sweetness (fructose or sugar) in the plantain to acid - not just acid, but concentrated acid. Lopsam went further to say that many disease conditions are traceable to the acid content in the body. In fact, acid has been identified as the cause of most of the body pains we experience. She, therefore, advised that we should steer clear of acid-forming foods, because they are extremely dangerous if we want to enjoy good health and live long. She also noted that even though foods like beans are acid-forming, during metabolism, such acid is called pH balance (acid alkaline balance), adding that this is good, provided your body can digest it well.

What Lopsam is saying in essence is that, during metabolism of protein foods, the hydrochloric acid in the stomach and the proteases enzyme break them down to smaller chains of amino acids, while at the same time the pancreas releases enzymes and bicarbonate buffer, an alkaline that goes to reduce the acidity of the digested food. This is a kind of neutralization reaction.

Lopsam also revealed that foods become poison to the body when they are damaged by fire and improperly combined, and that it is the liver that suffers the consequences. The problem here is that beans takes between 5 to7 hours to digest properly before leaving the stomach, while plantain takes 3 hours to digest. Moreover, while fruits digest in the terminal ileum, beans digest in the stomach. Also, ripe plantain does not need pancreatic enzyme to digest but beans needs pancreatic enzyme to digest. So, when both are combined, the ripe plantain tries to leave the stomach for the terminal ileum where its digestion is supposed to take place, but the beans will not allow it. This struggle goes on for a long period, until fermentation begins to take place. As you may know, fermentation in the stomach is a major source of many known diseases today. Therefore, combining beans and fried ripe plantain is a delicious poison, and as such she advised that we avoid cooking, baking, frying, and boiling ripe plantain. It is best to eat it raw. She added very importantly however that it is pertinent to note that good health cannot be achieved by luck but by implicit obedience to God's divine laws and health laws.

Building Blocks of Protein

Recall that it was earlier noted that the protein foods we eat are broken down into amino acids. There are 20 known amino acids, and they are the building blocks of proteins. These amino acids are: Arginine, leucine, isoleucine, alanine, phenylalanine, valine, tyrosine, proline, glutamine, serine, glycine, cysteine, lysine, threonine, histidine, methionine, tryptophan, aspartic acid, asparagine, glutamic acid.

Eight of these 20 amino acids are designated and characterized as essential amino acids, because our body cannot produce them; we depend on the food we eat to nourish our body with these eight amino acids, which are: methionine, lysine, valine, tryptophan, leucine, isoleucine, threonine and phenylalanine. Deficiency of any one of the 20 known amino acids will lead to disease conditions, which may be catastrophic.

Note however, that plant protein is not complete protein because plants do not have all the 20 amino acids in them. Animal protein is complete protein because it contains all the 20 amino acids. Therefore, you cannot depend on plant protein alone to get all the amino acids your body needs.

In conclusion, lipids consist of natural fats and oils. They are insoluble in water and form emulsion with dilute alkalis. During metabolism, fats and oils are broken down into fatty acids and glycerol before they are assimilated into the body. We also have essential fatty acids, which the body cannot produce and must be obtained from food sources. These essential fatty acids are linoleic acid and arachidonic acid. The function of lipids is to activate enzymes contained in the mitochondrion and form part of the electron transport system in the mitochondrion, which is covered in a medium of phospholipids (cell membrane). The mitochondrion is the powerhouse of the cell. This is where energy is generated, and as such, care must be taken to prevent the entrance of any foreign agent or substance into our body, because this is capable of causing a disruption of the integrity of the inner mitochondria membrane, and this will bring about disorders in the system.

CHAPTER THREE

PLANTS AND THEIR HEALTH BENEFITS

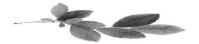

Nature, the way God designed it, is remarkably interesting and dynamic. Part of the many dynamics of nature is that the products of excretion in plants are, in most cases, the actual health benefits that humans derive from plants. These excretory products are formed because of respiration and metabolic activities taking place in the plant cells and are stored in the leaves, fruits, bark, stem, roots, sepals, and flowers. Examples of these excretory products are glycosides, tannins, alkaloids, plant oils, digitalis, sarsaparilla, anthocyanin pigments, morphine, quinine, cocaine, cinnamon, eucalyptus, turpentine, camphor, latex, gums, mucilage's, resins, etc.

Apart from the waste products of plants listed above, plants also have water, oxygen , and carbon dioxide as their excretory products. These products are also incredibly significant in the life of humans, as carbon dioxide is required in the process of photosynthesis. For all these to happen, the plants themselves require a good amount of nutrients to develop adequately to avoid any form of deficiency or stunted growth.

Mineral Elements and Vitamins

There are many plant products that are required by humans for healthy living. Among these are the mineral elements, such as sodium, potassium, calcium, magnesium, zinc, iron, manganese, copper, phosphorus, carbon, nitrogen, hydrogen, and other anti-inflammatory and antioxidant properties.

Only about 20 of all the naturally occurring elements are bountifully supplied to us in our natural food. Yet even this is dependent on whether they are not lost or destroyed during meal preparation, processing, or by way of improper food handling.

Many symptoms, disease conditions, contaminated food or improper food handling have been traced to deficiency of these mineral elements and vitamins.

Glycoside, Glucose and Alkaloids

The excretory products of plants, as previously mentioned, are divided into three categories: glycoside, because they contain sugar; glucoside, because they contain glucose; and alkaloids, because they contain nitrogenous compounds that are poisonous to insects, which the plants use as defensive mechanism against insects.

Glycoside is digitalis, which is obtained from foxglove plants. It is used in the treatment of heart diseases. It can also be used to increase the flow of blood throughout the body. But it is not safe for self-medication. You must use based on your doctor's advice. Sarsaparilla is obtained from smilax (herbaceous). It is used in the treatment of Psoriasis, arthritis, syphilis, cancer, gonorrhea. It is used by drinking the tea made from sarsaparilla roots. It is also used in the treatment of liver disease and to protect the liver from damage. Sarsaparilla can be combined with other herbs to facilitate their quick absorption into the system.

Note that only sarsaparilla from the smilax plant can be used. It should not be mistaken for the Indian sarsaparilla (Hemidesmus indicus), as this does not have the same active chemical with the former.

Tannins are obtained from the cell sap, cell wall and in the dead tissues of trees, like chestnuts, conifers, mangroves, and oaks, and in some cases, the tea leaves, and fruits. Some of these tannins are glucosides. Tannins are also found in spices, nuts, seeds, and leguminous plants. They are the defense mechanism against pests. They are used to color and add flavor to food and drinks. Tannins lower blood pressure, lower blood lipid level, facilitate blood clotting and produce liver necrosis and control immune responses.

In the alkaloids group, the morphine obtained from the opium poppy plant (Papaver somniferum), is used to treat acute and chronic pain. It works by releasing the neurotransmitter in the brain, called dopamine, thereby blocking the pain signals from reaching the brain and creating pleasant feeling in the patient. When not safely used according to a physician's advice, it can cause a side-effect known as dependence, which leads to addiction.

Specific Health Benefits of Plants

We will now consider various plants and their health benefits.

➢ **Quinine** is obtained from the Cinchona tree and it is used in the treatment of malaria. It does not prevent malaria but kills the plasmodium parasite responsible for malaria. You can boil the bark of cinchona tree in water to extract quinine locally, but it should be taken in moderation to avoid side effects like bleeding, allergic reactions, irregular heartbeat, and kidney damage.

➢ **Cocaine** is obtained from the coca plant. It is used medically as an anesthetic because it blocks nerve impulses, specifically the norepinephrine uptake, causing vasoconstriction in the arteries and vasculature in the splanchnic area and anesthesia. This procedure is carried out only by the doctor. Cocaine is a dangerous drug and should be avoided. It can trigger a whole lot of bad health conditions, especially increased blood pressure and increased heartbeat, which can result in heart attack and stroke; therefore, it is unsafe to use it. The leaves of the coca plant are used for the preparation of tea to increase brain functions and general activities. The tea is also used for the treatment of altitude sickness, for people who are afraid of heights. But this is only in places like the Peruvian Andes and not in a place like the United States, where it is considered a contraband.

➢ **Cinnamon** is obtained from the cinnamon tree. There are two types: Ceylon cinnamon and Cassia cinnamon. The more commonly known one is the Ceylon cinnamon. It is used as an anti-inflammatory agent. It enhances insulin sensitivity, reduces the level of sugar in the blood, and combats Alzheimer's and Parkinson's diseases. It also combats the HIV virus, bacteria, and fungi infections, and defends the body against cancer. Cinnamon is greatly beneficial to health, especially the Ceylon cinnamon. If you are using the Cassia cinnamon, ensure to use a small portion of it per time as it has a harmful effect, when taken in large quantity.

➢ **Camphor** is obtained from camphor tree. There are different types of camphor: those used topically and those that can be eaten. Edible camphor is used for the treatment of digestive issues, cold (cough) and asthma. It enhances blood circulation, triggers hormones, and takes care of muscle spasms. It is quite easy to use; all you need to do is to put it in warm water and drink. The non-edible camphor is used for treating fungus and eczema. It also enhances hair growth and kills head lice. It can also reduce pain and swelling on the skin.

> **Eucalyptus** is obtained from the eucalyptus tree. The leaves of eucalyptus tree, when dried, can be used to make tea, which is potent in reducing the risk of dementia, heart disease and cancer. It is also used for the treatment of cold and nasal congestion, cough, and associated headache. The oil is used to treat sinus congestion and it is a good mosquito repellent etc.

> **Turpentine** is obtained from the pine tree. The leaves, called the pine needle, can be used to make tea, which contains a good amount of vitamins A and C. The tea can reduce high blood pressure and treat heart disease. It should, however, not be taken by pregnant women. Moreover, one must ensure that what is being taken is pine needle, because there are other plants which resemble the pine needle, like the yew and cypress. These two are extremely dangerous and should not be mistaken for pine needle leaves.

> **Cannabidiol (CBD)** oil is extracted from marijuana or hemp cannabis plant. This oil does not have the capacity to make one high as marijuana does. It can be used in the treatment of epilepsy (seizure), migraines, depression, rheumatoid arthritis, cancer, acne, pain, autism, multiple sclerosis, and post-traumatic stress disorder (PTSD). Also, it reduces the rate of development of Alzheimer's disease, reduces anxiety, treats glaucoma, attention deficit/hyperactivity disorder (ADHD), and attention deficit disorder (ADD) - that is, it helps to have better cognitive performance and concentration, thereby

promoting focus and precision in handling task at hand.

CBD oil prevents and regulates diabetes and improves the capacity of lung function. The cannabis genus comprises many species which include, cannabis sativa, cannabis indica, and cannabis ruderalis, which originated in Central Asia. Cannabidiol (CBD) was discovered in the 1940s and in 2018, clinical research on it showed its medical significance when it was used experimentally on the study of pain, movement disorders, cognitive function, and anxiety. When CBD oil is obtained from hemp cannabis plant and contains less than 0.3 percent of Tetrahydrocannabinol (THC) it will not make people experience high sensations that put them in a state of euphoria. But when CBD oil is extracted from the marijuana cannabis plants, it usually has a higher concentration of Tetrahydrocannabinol (THC) which makes people to experience high sensations that put them in a state of euphoria. THC is the active ingredient or the psychoactive compound in marijuana that makes people feel high, which is why it is considered a hard drug. Both THC and CBD interact with the body's endocannabinoid system but produce different effects. The side effects of THC are dry mouth, red eyes, memory loss, slower reaction times, lack of coordination and increased heartbeat, even though it is good for treatment of muscle spasm, pain, nausea, glaucoma, low appetite, insomnia, and anxiety. The CBD oil does not have any recorded side effects, only that it may interact with the other medication in the system; that is, CBD to medication interaction.

➢ **Asparagus officinalis** belongs to the genus asparagus. It is a flowering plant species. The shoots of it are generally used as a spring vegetable. The plant originated in Europe (northern Spain). It produces a red berry fruit that is poisonous to humans; but the shoots are of great benefit, as they are loaded with minerals like folate, iron, calcium, and vitamins, like vitamin A, E, and K. The plant contains a high level of protein, known as histones. Histones contribute actively in controlling cell growth. They are low in calories and a great source of mineral nutrients, including fiber.

➢ **Asparagus** is known to lower blood pressure and improve digestion. It is good to eat it during pregnancy, as it helps you experience a healthy pregnancy and smooth delivery. Asparagus is loaded with nutrients, and it is best eaten raw. This does not mean that you cannot cook it to get your desired flavor of it. A cup of asparagus, when cooked, contains about 4 grams of protein, fiber and up to 404 milligrams of potassium. Potassium is good for blood pressure and contains asparaptine that helps to improve blood flow.

➢ **Avocado** is known to possess a high level of nutrients and health benefits. It is a good source of vitamin C, E, K and B-6, as well as riboflavin, niacin, folate pantothenic acid, magnesium, and potassium. It also has antioxidant properties. It is full of good fats, which are beneficial to health because of their ability to lower "bad" cholesterol levels. This means that it can lower the body's Low-Density Lipoprotein (LDL) bad cholesterol and increase the High-Density Lipoprotein (HDL) good cholesterol.

In whatever form you want to eat it, either as guacamole or mixed with salad, you are sure of getting the health benefits. Avocado protects the eyes, as it contains carotenoid and the antioxidant known as lutein, which plays a key role in eye health. Because of its health benefits, avocado is used to enhance good heart health, helps lower blood pressure, helps reverse insulin resistance, has anti-aging properties, helps maintain bowel function, and helps reduce the risk of Alzheimer's. It can also reduce stomach inflammation, may aid stroke prevention, and may also increase the level of lutein, which protects against muscular degeneration. Avocado is a fruit that attacks diabetes and prevents stroke.

➢ **Apple** belongs to the genus Malus plant family and it originated from central Asia. The ancestor of apple, Malus sieversii, is still cultivated in central Asia to date, but has gone into extinction in other parts of the world. Apple is a sweet, edible fruit that is cultivated worldwide. Apples are extraordinarily rich in antioxidants, dietary fiber, and flavonoids. The phytonutrients and antioxidants in apples may help reduce the risk of developing cancer, hypertension, diabetes, and heart disease. Little wonder it gained the slogan, "an apple a day, keeps the doctor away." Apples protect your heart, prevent constipation, block diarrhea, improve lung cancer, cushion joints, and brighten the eyes. Apples must be eaten regularly to get the desired health benefits. Note, however, that the seeds of apples are poisonous, as they contain a high level of cyanide.

➢ **Lemongrass** is botanically known as Cymbopogon citratus or Andropogon flexuous. The leaves and oil are commonly used to prepare herbal medicine. Lemongrass is usually taken orally but sometimes applied to the skin when squeezed. It helps to prevent the growth of some bacteria and yeast. It contains some substances that are believed to relieve pain and swelling. It reduces fever and lowers cholesterol level in the blood. It also stimulates the uterus and enhances menstrual flow.

Investigation suggests that drinking lemongrass tea decreases the symptoms of thrush (yeast infection in the mouth) in people with HIV/AIDS. It is used for stomach and intestinal cramp, convulsion in children, vomiting, diabetes, headaches, rheumatism, etc. The health benefits of lemongrass are numerous, but the following are of great significance: It Cleanses the kidney, liver, pancreas, digestive tract and bladder; it kills cancer cells, and is a good anti-oxidant; it is used to treat blood pressure, flu and cold; it is a powerful detoxifier and effective pain killer; it is great for treating gout, fever, stress, indigestion; it is efficient for losing weight, and treats diarrhea and stomach ache. Besides, it is antibacterial and antifungal. To use, just boil it in water and drink it at regular intervals.

> **Broccoli** is a good source of vitamin C, folate, potassium, and fiber. The presence of vitamin C enables broccoli to build collagen, which forms the body tissues and bones. It also facilitates the healing of wounds. It is a well-known fact that vitamin C is a powerful antioxidant and protects the body from damaging free radicals.

Broccoli belongs to the vegetable family known as cruciferous vegetables. A wide variety of this family includes kale, cauliflower, Brussels sprouts, bok choy, cabbage, collard greens, rutabaga, and turnip. The health benefits of eating broccoli include fighting cancer, particularly lung and colon cancer; improving bone health; protecting from chronic diseases, owing to its high fiber content; lowering the risk of coronary heart disease, stroke, hypertension, diabetes, obesity and other gastrointestinal diseases.

Frequent intake of broccoli has been known to reduce blood pressure and cholesterol levels; as well as improving insulin sensitivity and promoting weight loss in overweight and obese people. Broccoli is known to improve digestion and prevent constipation. It improves the immune system and reduces inflammation. Although broccoli has been notoriously believed not to be most people's favorite, its reputation as one of the healthiest vegetables is undeniably true. Eat broccoli to live long and enjoy life.

➢ **Aloe Vera** is grown almost everywhere for its health benefits. It is used as an antibacterial agent. It facilitates the healing of burns and reduces dental plaque. It is used in the treatment of canker sores, lowers blood sugar levels, treats constipation, improves skin health, and prevents wrinkles.

➢ **Garlic**, as studies have shown, is an effective natural antibiotic and becomes more powerful when eaten raw on an empty stomach. It is advisable that you eat garlic before breakfast, as bacteria are more vulnerable in the morning. In herbal medicine, garlic is highly effective in the treatment of many illnesses, like high blood pressure and heart diseases. It helps the bladder and liver to function properly. It can cure stomach problems like diarrhea. It also stimulates appetite and digestion. It is not a surprise that garlic is considered a healing food and it is known all over the world.

Another amazing fact is that garlic can cure respiratory diseases, detoxify the body, cure depression, diabetes, typhus, and some kinds of cancers. Garlic can remove worms and parasites from the system. It can cure and prevent pneumonia, asthma, chronic bronchial catarrhs, bronchitis, tuberculosis and more.

In the case of tuberculosis, it is advised that you eat a whole bulb of garlic a day. It should be eaten raw or slightly browned. To help better the taste, you can make a sauce of garlic with oil and egg yolk. You can also mash and mixed with honey and take raw.

A solution of garlic can be prepared by collecting 200 grams of garlic, 1000 grams of water, 700 grams of refined sugar. Boil the water, mash the garlic, add honey to it, and take three table spoons a day for bronchial problems.

Garlic also cures earaches, constipation, hemorrhoids, and toothache. Take a little garlic juice and then apply 1 or 2 drops into the painful ear. In case of hemorrhoids and constipation, boil water with garlic, put the solution into a container, then breathe in the vapor from the container.

➤ **Onion** contains a lot of vitamins, with antioxidant and antibacterial properties. Onion has the following health benefits:

o Improves immunity

o Regulates blood sugar

o Anti-Inflammatory

o Antiseptic

o Remedy for common cold, cough, fever and sore throat

o Reduces pain

o Prevents tooth decay

o Eliminates worms in the stomach

o Eliminates hair lice when applied to the hair

o Prevents allergies.

➢ **Star fruit** contains analgesic, anti-inflammatory, hypotension, anthelmintic, antioxidant, anti-ulcer, hypocholesterolemic, hypolipidemic, antimicrobial, antimicrobial, anti-tumor properties. It is used in the treatment of diabetes, lowers cholesterol level, reduces the risk of stroke, and heart disease. It is also rich in vitamin B and C.

➢ **Pomegranate** contains fiber, protein, folate, potassium, vitamin C, and vitamin K. It prevents arthritis, fights erectile dysfunction, improves memory, lowers blood pressure, helps in digestion, boosts immunity, prevents plaque formation in the mouth, helps in digestion, thins the blood, protects from free radicals, prevents atherosclerosis, prevents blood clot, helps blood to flow freely, improves oxygen level in the body, and prevents cancer and stroke. It also has anti-aging properties.

➢ **Kiwi** is a high source of vitamin C and dietary fiber. It contains an enzyme called actinidain that resembles the enzyme papain of papaya, both of which are used to tenderize meat. It is a good source of potassium.

Consumption of kiwi can lower the risk of cardiovascular disease (CVD) and coronary heart disease (CHD) due to its high fiber content. Kiwi also controls blood pressure, cholesterol, and blood sugar levels. It is a good source of folate, which is beneficial for pregnant women, as it helps in the development of fetus. It also protects DNA from damaging.

➤ **Soursop** contains thiamine, magnesium, potassium, vitamin C, protein, fiber, carbohydrates, and some calories. It is a natural cancer killer, which is more effective than chemotherapy. The soursop leaves tea helps to refurbish the nerves and treat insomnia.

➤ **Mangosteen's** extract contains antioxidant, antitumoral, antiallergic, anti-inflammatory, antibacterial, and antiviral properties. It can cause cell death in Leukemia cells (cancer of the white blood cell). It is good for the treatment of diarrhea, dysentery, infected wounds, abdominal pain, suppuration, and chronic ulcer. Xanthones have also been isolated from the pericarp, fruit, heartwood, and leaves.

➤ **Loganberry** is acidic in nature. It is used for the prevention of common cold, constipation, flu, gout, stress, anxiety, fatigue, depression, and cancer of any kind. It promotes brain health, healthy heart, good digestion, tissue development, bones and nervous system development and has antimicrobial properties. It fights muscular degeneration, strengthens immune system, helps in weight loss, reduces wrinkles, and can be used as antidote for snake bite.

> **Papaya** originated from Central America and Southern Mexico. Its botanical name is Carica papaya and is also known as pawpaw in other countries. It grows very well in tropical regions. The leaves of papaya plants are used to tenderize meat (makes meat soft).

Papaya Health Benefits

o Rich in Vitamin C
o Fights infection
o Gets rid of free radicals, since Vitamin C is an antioxidant
o Rich in Vitamin A, which is good for eyesight. Keeps your skin and mucous membranes healthy.
o Useful in fighting macular degeneration
o It has folate, riboflavin, thiamin, and pyridoxine, all of which are vitamins that our body requires but cannot produce. When you eat papaya daily, you will get a good supply of these vitamins.

Papaya also cures sicknesses, such as heart disease, rheumatoid arthritis, and atherosclerosis. It can strengthen the immune system and boost digestive health, which ultimately helps in keeping your overall wellbeing. Papaya has flavonoids, such as beta-carotene, and studies have revealed that beta-carotene can help protect the body against the formation of certain cancers, especially mouth and lung cancers.

It also has flavonoid zeaxanthin, cryptoxanthin, and

Lutein, which have potent antioxidant compounds that remove free radicals. All these antioxidants can work together to prevent premature aging, as well as degenerative diseases. Whether you consume ripe or unripe papaya, you will surely get the benefit. It also cures stomach ulcer.

➢ **Banana** contains high amount of potassium. Eating banana daily helps to lower blood pressure and lessen the possibility of atherosclerosis, heart attack and stroke. Banana aids in calcium absorption and contains high level of fructooligosaccharide (FOS) that promotes calcium absorption. FOS nourishes healthy bacteria in the colon and boosts the body's ability to absorb nutrients. It prevents muscle cramps, helps maintain low blood sugar, has vitamin B6, and helps with nerve functions.

➢ **Cantaloupe** is a good source of potassium, which is responsible for lowering blood pressure and keeping the electrical activity of the heart stable. Cantaloupe juice helps to maintain the right electrolyte balance, and hydrates the body, which prevent dryness and itchiness of the skin. It protects the heart, delays the signs of aging, and enhances your vision or eyesight.

➢ **Ripe bananas with black spots on yellow skin** produce a substance called tumor necrosis factor (TNF). It could fight abnormal cells in the body. The more the black spots, the better, because it has immunity-boosting quality. Also, the riper the banana, the better the anti-cancer quality.

➢ **Bitter kola** is biologically known as **Garcinia kola**, and it belongs to the family of Guittiferae. Its medicinal value includes the treatment of:

- o Osteoarthritis
- o Glaucoma (eye pressure)
- o HIV
- o Cold
- o Male infertility (impotence)
- o Food poison
- o Ebola

It is also used to detoxify the body system

➢ **Bryophyllum leaf:** This plant is native to South Africa and Madagascar. There are about forty species in the group.

Health Benefits:

1. Used for the treatment of cough: The juice is extracted by heating it on fire for about 5 minutes to soften the leaf. Then squeeze the juice out of it and add little quantity of salt before drinking. You can also chew it or make tea with it.

2. It is used for the treatment of diabetes, asthma, cold, constipation, boil, and high blood pressure (HBP). It is also used for the treatment of piles (hemorrhoids),

bloody diarrhea, jaundice, and many other ailments. The rhizome of the bryophyllum can be used as a preventive measure for kidney stone.

➤ **Beets** are greatly beneficial in the treatment of anemia, indigestion, constipation pile, kidney disorders, dandruff, gallbladder disorders, cancer, and heart diseases. They also help to prevent macular degeneration, improve blood circulation, aid skin care, prevent cataracts, and treat respiration problems. These benefits of beetroots can be attributed to their richness in nutrients, vitamins and minerals, magnesium, iron, copper, phosphorous and being a good source of flavonoids called anthocyanins. They have low calories, with no cholesterol, but they have the highest sugar content of all vegetables, and therefore, should be eaten moderately.

Beets have been implicated as an aphrodisiac or sexual booster for a long time. This is because beets contain a good level of the mineral boron, which is known to boost the production of sexual hormones. This can lead to a boost in libido, thereby increasing fertility, sperm mobility improvement, and a reduction in frigidity in the bedroom. Your sexual life can get a legitimate, time-tested push in the right direction by adding beets to your diet. Beets also boost energy.

➤ **Moringa oleifera** is the ultimate super food. It has 90 different types of nutrients, which are vitamins, proteins, fiber, minerals, 46 antioxidants, 36 anti-inflammatory agents, 18 amino acids and 9 essential amino acids.

➢ **Bermudagrass (Cynodon dactylon**) is anti-viral and anti-microbial. It is used for stomach ailment, wounds, piles, eczema, eye problems, skin rashes, constipation/indigestion, mental debility, diabetes, epilepsy, vaginal problems, menstrual problems, kidney liver problems, acidity ulcer, colitis, and stomach pain. It reduces acidity and increases alkalinity. It is also good for urinary tract infection. It promotes regular bowel movement and helps to remove phlegm from the body. It also helps to stop nose bleeding. It strengthens teeth and bones. Cynodon dactylon is very refreshing when mixed with turmeric and lemon. Just blend the grass, sieve out the juice, and then drink it.

➢ **Lecithin** is great for mobilization of fats. It is derived from sunflower seeds, soy products, cottonseed, and canola. Lecithin helps to reduce the bad cholesterol LDL in the body and at the same time helps to increase the good cholesterol HDL in the body. Lecithin helps the body to distribute its weight equally. Excess muscle and fats are taken from the parts of the body where they are in excess and transferred to the parts where they are low or absent. Lecithin is an emulsifying agent that causes fats to dissolve and remain in solution.

Regular intake of lecithin will keep the cholesterol from sedimentation and deposition in the arterial walls. Lecithin can dissolve even the cholesterol that has already been deposited in the walls. It is exceptionally good for the cardiovascular system; in that it increases your vigor and vitality.

➢ **Cashew leaves and bark** extract is used to reduce blood sugar and high blood pressure levels, as well as internal heat. The extract is obtained from boiling the leaves in water. It is good for the formation of red blood cells, in case of sickle cell anemia. It is also used to treat heart disease, nerves, and muscle functions, gallstones, and diabetes. The extract is high in antioxidants, good for immune system support. It is good for people undergoing tumor and cancer treatment and bone health. Decoction prepared from cashew leaves and the bark of the tree is used for treatment of diarrhea and thrush.

➢ **Allamanda plant** is used to treat liver disease, skin disease, reduce swelling and kill bacteria. It is also used to neutralize free radicals.

➢ **Cassava - Manihot utilissima (bitter cassava), Manihot palmata (sweet cassava) or Manihot esculenta (Yucca root)** is particularly good in the treatment of arthritis, fever, headache, and boosts immunity. It has antioxidant properties and boosts cell regeneration. The leaves and stem can be boiled very well to allow some of the water evaporate and then allow it cool down before drinking. The leaves are also good for making soup.

➢ **Pride of Barbados (Caesalpinia Pulcherrima)** is used for the treatment of fever. Prepare an infusion of the flowers, use it two times daily. In the case of menstrual abnormalities, make a decoction of the leaves and take it twice daily for a period of about two weeks.

➢ **Waterleaf plant (Talinum Triangulare)** is called *gbologi* (in Etsako language, Edo State, Nigeria). Other parts of Edo State call it *ebedondon*. In Yoruba language, it is called *gbure*. It is used in treatment of blood clotting (Thrombosis) and general improvement of the entire body system. It is used to improve cerebral hypo perfusion, schizophrenia and prevent death of the brain cells.

➢ **Euphorbia hirta,** sometimes called asthma-plant **(Tawa Tawa)** is called *ewe emile* in Yoruba language, Nigeria. It is used for the treatment of asthma. All you need to do is to get the leaves, flowers, and roots, and make soup or stew with it. Eat it twice daily, or as needed.

➢ **Milk bush (Sehund plant)** is good for the treatment of the following ailments:

  o Cough: Heat up the leaves on fire and squeeze them to extract the juice, add salt and drink twice daily, for two weeks.

  o Tooth extraction: Extract the milk and drop it on the affected tooth to loosen it for easy removal. Ensure that the milk does not touch another tooth.

o Ear pain: Heat up the extracted milk and add two drops to the affected ear; it will eradicate the pain.

o Muscle swelling: Extract the milk and apply it to the area that is swollen. It will bring down the stiffness and swelling.

o Toothache: Soak cotton wool in the milk, burn it, then put the burnt cotton wool on affected tooth. It will treat the toothache.

o Intestinal worms: Make a paste of the root of milk bush, with asafetida and apply the paste on the stomach. It kills intestinal worms, especially in children.

o Ulcers: Blend the leaves, Indian beech, and jasmine in cow's urine; apply the paste to the ulcer or boils externally.

o Boils and moles on skin: These are eruptions on the skin. Extract the milk and apply to the eruption; it will treat and clear the skin.

o Psoriasis: Extract the juice and add equal quantity of mustard oil, cook it, and then rub it on the affected area.

o Eye pain: Extract the juice and mix it with the ash of sweet oil, dry it under the sun to form powder, and use it as eyeliner.

CHAPTER FOUR

THE NATURE OF DISEASES

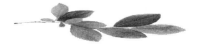

Diseases are caused by germs and the main infecting agents are bacteria, fungi, and viruses. These germs find their way into the body through contaminated food, water, air, cuts on the skin, animal and insect bites, and droplets from body fluid and mucous membrane.

Some diseases caused by bacteria are tetanus, diphtheria, meningitis, whooping cough, tuberculosis, plague, typhoid fever, dysentery, syphilis, cholera, gonorrhea, pneumonia, gastroenteritis, botulism, boil, etc. Those caused by fungi are ringworm, athlete's foot, a kind of meningitis, superficial candidiasis, intestinal candidiasis, and a host of human allergies, etc. And those caused by viruses are swine fever/flu, cowpox, fowl pest, rabies, poliomyelitis, yellow fever, smallpox, influenza, measles, coronavirus, etc.

The actions of these organisms result in the malfunctioning of the various organs, depending on whether the disease is localized or systemic in nature. Other abnormal disease conditions are caused by inflammation, environmental factors and genetic defects, which are characterized by different signs and symptoms. Some of these diseases are of significant concern, as their devastations on human lives and livelihoods, through epidemics and pandemics, have, at different times, changed the course of history.

Chronicles of Plagues and Pandemics

There have been series of epidemics and pandemics, dating back to the prehistoric era and stretching into modern times. For example, the **prehistoric epidemic** of circa 3000 B.C consumed an entire village in China and all the inhabitants of the village were burnt to stop the spread of the disease. The **plague of Athens** in 430 B.C. ravaged the people of Athens and Sparta and took the lives of approximately 100,000 people. The **Antonine plague** of A.D. 165-180, killed over 5 million people in the Roman Empire.

The **Plague of Cyprian**, Bishop of Carthage (A.D. 250-271), was estimated to have killed 5,000 people a day only in Rome, excluding other places. The **Plague of Justinian** (A.D. 541-542) ravaged the Byzantine Empire by the bubonic plague and 10% of the world's population was estimated to have died. The **Black Death** of 1346-1353, killed half of Europe's population and left devastation in its wake, as it traveled from Asia to Europe and other parts of the world. The **Cocoliztli epidemic** of 1545-1548, was a kind of viral hemorrhagic fever that caused the death of 15 million inhabitants of Mexico and Central America, amidst extreme drought that had already weakened the population. It was utterly catastrophic.

The **American plagues** of the 16th century caused the collapse of the Inca and Aztec civilizations and wiped out 90% of the inhabitants of the Western Hemisphere. The disease weakened the Aztec and the Incan armies and made it easy for the Spanish forces to conquer the territories of both empires. The **Great Plague of London** (1665-1666), caused a mass exodus from London and by the end of the plague, about 100,000 people, including 15% of the population of London, had died. The **Great Plague of Marseille** (1720-1723), claimed the lives of about 100,000 people within the space of three years in the city of Marseille in France and surrounding areas. It was estimated that 30% of the inhabitant of Marseille may had died.

The **Russian Plague** of 1770-1772, swept across Moscow and left about 100,000 people dead. The quarantined citizens took to violence, when they could no longer bear the terror of the ravaging plague. The riot that followed, spread throughout the city of Moscow, and led to the gruesome murder of Archbishop Ambrosius, who was working assiduously to sensitize the crowds not to gather for worship.

The **Philadelphia Yellow Fever Epidemic** of 1793 claimed the lives of more than 5,000 people in Philadelphia and was transmitted by mosquitoes, which increased greatly in number due to the hot and humid summer weather that was favorable for their breeding. The epidemic finally stopped in the wake of the winter season that killed all the mosquitoes.

The **Flu Pandemic** of 1889-1890 wreaked havoc, which spanned the entire world. Within a few months, it had killed 1 million people. Even though air movement did not exist at the time, the virus spread rapidly throughout Europe and the rest of the world, taking just five weeks to reach its peak mortality. The **American Polio Epidemic** of 1916 occurred sporadically in the United States and caused the death of 6,000 people. Poliomyelitis is also known as infantile paralysis because it affects mainly children below age five and leaves those that survive with permanent disabilities. It was the development of the Salk vaccine in 1954 that reduced the spread of the disease.

The **Spanish Flu** of 1918-1920, affected approximately 500 million people around the region of the South Seas to the North Pole and claimed the lives of one-fifth of the affected people. Some communities were pushed to the brink of extinction. Despite the name, however, history has it that the flu did not breakout in Spain.

The **Asian flu** of 1957-1958 originated in China and caused a worldwide pandemic, which claimed the lives of more than 1 million people. The virus that caused the pandemic was a characteristic blend of avian flu viruses. The disease spread rapidly and stretched into Singapore, Hong Kong, and the coastal cities of the United States, in the wake of the summer of 1957. The total death toll recorded worldwide was more than 1.1 million, with 116,000 deaths recorded in the United States.

The **Acquired Immune Deficiency Syndrome (AIDS)** pandemic of 1981 to present day has claimed over 35 million lives, since it was first recognized. Records have it that the Human Immunodeficiency Virus, which causes AIDS, may have developed from a chimpanzee's virus that was transmitted to humans in West Africa in the 1920s. The virus swept across the world, causing a devastating pandemic by the outset of the 20th century. Out of the estimated 40 million people living with HIV, 64% are living in the sub-Saharan Africa. Even though there is no known cure for HIV/AIDS, medication has been developed that now allows people with the disease to lead normal lives with regular treatment.

The **H1N1 swine flu pandemic** of 2009-2010, originated in Mexico in the spring of 2009 before spreading to other parts of the world. The death toll of the flu was between 151,700 and 575,400 according to the Centers for Disease Control and Prevention (CDC) and the total number of infected people was 1.4 billion people worldwide. The virus affected mainly children and young adults, and 80% of deaths recorded were of people below the age of 65, according to CDC reports. This pandemic lasted close to two years.

The H1N1 virus had similar characteristics with the influenza virus and was first identified in 2009. Even though the H1N1 flu originated in Mexico, the first case (person infected) in the United States was discovered in California on April 15th, 2009 and the second case was discovered on

April 17th, 2009 about 130 miles away from the first person infected without any prior contact, relationship, association or connection with the first person infected. On April 23rd, 2009 two more cases of people infected with the H1N1 virus, were detected in Texas, which resulted in an investigation into interstates outbreak and response.

The virus went further to cause a worldwide pandemic and continued through April of 2010 and beyond, with series of research, investigation, treatment, vaccination and infection control going on, so that between April 2009 and April 2010, the CDC held 60 related media events, 39 press briefings and 22 tele-briefings, which reached more than 35,000 participants. On August 11th, 2010, the World Health Organization (WHO) announced the end of 2009 H1N1 Swine Flu Pandemic.

The **West African Ebola epidemic** ravaged some African countries from 2014-2016. There were 28,600 cases of infected people and 11,325 deaths. The first case was discovered in December of 2013 in Guinea, after which the disease hurriedly spread to Liberia and Sierra Leone. Majority of the cases and deaths occurred in these countries, and a few numbers of cases were recorded in Senegal, Mali, Nigeria, Europe and the United States, according to reports by the CDC. The very first known cases of Ebola occurred in Sudan and the Democratic Republic of Congo in 1976 and it was said that the virus may have originated in bats.

There is also the **Zika virus epidemic** of 2015 to date.

This virus is usually transmitted by mosquitoes of the genus Aedes and through sexual intercourse in humans. The Aedes mosquitoes usually flourish best in warm, humid climates, which is why Central America, South America and the Southern parts of the United States are the prime areas for the virus to thrive. It was said that the impact of the Zika virus epidemic in South America and Central America may not be known for several years - the reason being that while the virus attacks infants who are still in the womb and causes birth defects, it is not harmful to adults or children. Scientists are still fighting to bring the Zika virus under control.

The **coronavirus pandemic** of 2019 (also known as COVID-19) to date, first showed up in Wuhan, China, in late December 2019. From there, it made its way into the United States in mid-January, causing the first death in the United States at the end of February. In the United States, over 3,576,430 million cases of infection and 138,360 deaths have been reported at the time of writing this book. Recent information revealed that COVID-19 may have appeared in the United States earlier than January, because an autopsy carried out on a Californian woman, who was diagnosed with the virus and died on the 6th of February, of what was assumed to be a heart attack, had actually revealed COVID-19. As at February 6th, it was already three weeks earlier than the previously reported first death case in the United States.

The danger posed by the coronavirus depends on the

characteristics of the virus, which includes how fast it spreads between people, the seriousness of the resulting sickness and measures available to control the impact of the virus, for example, medication, vaccines, and the relative success of the outcomes. The focus currently is on how to reduce the spread and impact of the COVID-19 virus worldwide.

Viruses are degenerate descendants of pathogenic microorganisms that are in the borderline or link between animate and inanimate matters. When introduced into a susceptible host, they can alter the activities of the host cells, in which they become established and elicit multiplication of themselves, to hundreds or even thousands of times the amount originally present. They are dangerous obligate parasites that are not visible to the naked eyes or ordinary light microscope. But with the use of an electron microscope, they become glaring. There are about seven or more properties associated with all the agents known as viruses, but only one will be mentioned here, and that is, all viruses exhibit definite tropism, which means that they are specific in their attack. They naturally attack one or a limited number of host species with a focus on specific tissues or cells within the host.

Food and living organisms generally provide an excellent medium for the growth of a variety of bacteria, viruses, and fungi, because of their nutritional content. Bacterial and viral diseases can be controlled by practicing hand washing, sterilizing food, and water, exterminating of animals that are the transmitting agents, proper sanitary conditions, good health habits or personal hygiene, and maintenance of body health.

Several medicinal plants have also been used to cure, prevent, and control some or most of these diseases and illnesses that affect man internally and externally. For example, water leaves (Talinum triangulare) which originated in West Africa and other parts of the world, have found their usefulness in the area of herbal medicine, for the treatment of high blood pressure, malaria, arthritis, anemia, insomnia, measles, diarrhea. Waterleaf is also known to improve blood clotting, weight loss, digestion, bones, and teeth. It aids in the treatment of infection/disease such as bacteria, fungi, and inflammatory diseases, and schizophrenia. Waterleaf also contains a lot of mineral nutrients like crude fiber, vitamin minerals, crude protein, and lipids.

CHAPTER FIVE

TREATMENT OF DISEASES

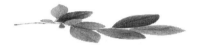

In this chapter, we will be considering different foods, plants, herbs, and how they can help in treatment of certain disease conditions.

Juices, Smoothies, Teas, and Their Benefits

CARROT JUICE: Blend a generous amount of carrots with water and then filter it to collect the juice.

It helps to:

1. Eliminate muscle aches and pain from physical exhaustion

2. Strengthen the lungs

3. Prevent heart attack

4. Strengthen immune system

5. Lessen menstrual pain

6. Prevent liver, kidney, and pancreas disease

7. Detoxify, assist with bowel movement, and eliminate constipation

8. To get clear eyesight

9. Prevent high blood pressure

10. Burn fat for weight loss

11. Prevent the development of cancer cells and stop their growth.

✓ TURMERIC SMOOTHIE:

1 cup of Coconut Milk

½ cup of frozen mango chunks

1 fresh banana

½ tbsp. of Turmeric

½ tbsp. of Cinnamon

½ tbsp. of ginger

½ tbsp. of chia seeds

Mix all of them together and blend into smoothie.

Health benefits:

1. Anti-inflammatory

2. Natural antibiotics

3. Prevents prostate cancer

4. Strengthens ligaments

5. Treats skin disorder

6. Cures cough

7. Prevents asthma

8. Reduces risk of colon cancer

9. Treats depression

10. Prevents Alzheimer's

11. Reduces arthritis

12. Detoxifies the liver

13. Blood purifier

14. Boosts metabolism

15. Antioxidant

16. Reduces risk of blood clots

17. Prevents stroke

18. Reduces bad cholesterol

19. Improves digestion

20. Slows the progression of multiple sclerosis.

✓ PINEAPPLE TEA

Get some pineapple peels, and boil in water for about 10 -15 minutes. Allow to cool down to room temperature and decant or filter. You can drink it hot or put the filtrate in the refrigerator and take it in portions daily with little honey, as needed.

✓ GREEN TEA

It prevents arthritis, treats Alzheimer's disease, strengthens bones, is anti-aging, prevents obesity, good for diabetes, prevents high blood pressure, prevents Parkinson's disease, good for liver diseases, boosts immune system and regulates blood sugar. It is also good for flu, prevents tooth decay and reduces stress, prevents food poisoning, and melts the fats in our body. It reduces cholesterol level, prevents heart diseases and stroke, facilitates recovery from heart attack, and reduces the risk of cancer growth.

✓ ANTIBIOTICS

To prepare antibiotics, use the following:

4 cups of apple cider vinegar

2/4 cups of garlic

2/4 cups of onions

3 fresh pepper

2/4 cups of ginger

2 ½ cups of horse radish soup

2 ½ cups of turmeric soup

3 ½ cups of honey.

Blend all these and mix; then pour apple cider vinegar to mix them properly. Place the container in a dark cool place for about 14 days, and then filter it by compression process. Drink a cup daily for 3 weeks.

Juice and smoothie blends that cure various ailments

1. Cold: Carrot, pineapple, ginger, garlic

2. Depression: Carrot, apple, spinach, beet

3. Headache: Apple, cucumber, kale, ginger, and celery

4. Diabetes: Carrot, spinach, and celery

5. Ulcer: Cabbage, carrot, celery, and papaya

6. Asthma: Carrot, spinach, apple, garlic, lemon

7. High Blood Pressure: Beet, apple, celery, cucumber, and ginger

8. Arthritis: Carrot, celery, pineapple, lemon

9. Kidney Detox: Carrot, watermelon, cucumber, and celery.

10. Kidney Stone: Orange, apple, Watermelon, Lemon

11. Eyes: Carrot, celery

12. Stress: Banana, strawberry, pear

13. Constipation: Carrots, apple, Fresh Cabbage

14. Fatigue: Carrots, beets, green apple, lemon, and spinach

15. Indigestion: Pineapple, carrot, lemon, and mint.

16. Memory Loss: Pomegranate, beet, and grapes

17. Hang over: Apple, carrot, beet, and lemon

Foods and fruits never to refrigerate

- Avocado
- Tomatoes
- Garlic
- Oil
- Cantaloupe
- Onions
- Bread
- Potatoes

Disease conditions and their herbal remedies

❖ **Sinus:** Break up thick mucus with a few drops of Eucalyptus or peppermint oil in hot water. With your face down over the water, drape a towel over the back of your neck and inhale the steam.

❖ **Cancer:** Take 1 beetroot, 1 Carrot, 1 apple, ½ lemon, 1 soursop, and blend together to make juice. If taken regularly, this juice can prevent cancer, heart attack, acne; it also strengthens immunity, eyes, liver, kidney, pancreas, and eliminates indigestion.

❖ **Puffy eyes**: Dip cotton balls in cold milk and place them on your eyes for about 15 minutes.

❖ **Internal ulcer**: Goat weed is a good herb for internal ulcer. Blend some of it with water and take a shot morning and evening for 2 weeks.

❖ **High blood pressure**: Take 4 lemons, 4 cloves of garlic, 2.5 inch of ginger peeled, blend together, boil in 2 liters of water and allow to cool, strain with a sieve, pour into a bottle, and keep in the refrigerator. Consume the remedy 2 hours before meal, twice daily. Shake the bottle very well before use as the ginger might settle at the bottom of the bottle. Another potent remedy for high blood pressure is a mixture of honey, ginger juice, and cumin powder. Mix 1 teaspoon of honey with 1 teaspoon ginger juice, 1 teaspoon cumin powder, and take them together twice a day. You can also get 4 seeds of English Pear (Avocado), cut them into pieces, dry under the sun and grind into powder. Put a teaspoon of this powder into your ready-to-drink pap; drink this once daily for 2 weeks.

❖ **Cough**: Get some lemons and squeeze the juice out of them, add a quantity of organic honey and olive oil. Bring the mixture to boil and allow this to cool down. Take ½ table spoon every 2 hours.

❖ **Diabetes**: Collect scent leaves or basil leaves (Ocimum americanum or Ocimum basilicum) and bitter leaves. Squeeze them together with warm water, add garlic and potash, or baking soda. Take 2 spoons, 3 times daily. You can also take two pieces of okra (lady finger) and cut both ends of each one. Put these two pieces in a glass of water, cover the glass and keep it at room temperature overnight. Early in the morning before breakfast, remove the okra from the glass of water and drink that water. Repeat this daily for about two weeks, and you will see a remarkable decrease in your blood sugar. You can also squeeze Siam weed leaves very well to get a glassful of it. Mix it with full cream milk, stir very well and drink it 3 times daily for 4 days a week. Repeat this for up to a month. Blend 6 bulbs of big onions; add one original bottle of honey. Take one spoon, 3 times a day for one month. Alternatively, get a handful of bitter leaf and scent leaves, squeeze out the juice in them, and add lime juice, garlic, and little quantity of potash. Take half a glass of it, 2 times daily for one month.

❖ **Malaria, epilepsy, and fever**: Get scent leaves (Basil Plant or Osmium species) and either squeeze out the juice and drink it or use it to make soup and drink it. Another effective way to treat malaria is to get lemongrass, unripe pineapple, ginger root and boil with water, allow it to cool down, filter it, and blend some garlic to it (when it has completely cooled down) take a glass cup, 3 times daily. For epilepsy, collect some passion flowers and passionflower leaves, put them in hot water, and add honey to it. Drink a glassful 3 times daily.

The following are also useful for the treatment of malaria, epilepsy, and fever:

- Cucumber helps to detoxify and purify the liver

- Pomegranate cleanse blood vessels

- Sweet potatoes balances hormones

- Papaya help to improve the absorption of nutrients into the bloodstream

- Turmeric helps to clean toxins from the liver

- Spinach cleans and strengthens the liver

- Broccoli helps to restore the liver

- Sprouts help the body absorb micronutrients

- Peaches nourishes the skin and digestive tract

- Bananas provide quick healing to the liver

- Celery juice helps to stabilize high and low blood pressure

- Ginger expels ammonia and toxins from the gut

- Apples starve out bacteria, yeast, and mold from our gut

- Lemons cleanse and purify the liver

- Cherries bind toxins in the liver and removes them, removes radiation from the body

- Figs removes toxins from the digestive tracts

- Kiwi helps dissolve gallstones

- Onions expels pathogens from the liver

- Apricots help to slow down aging process.

❖ **Constipation**: This is indigestion and issues associated with the gall bladder. Vegetable juices can help prevent or stop constipation. All you need to do is properly extract juice from fresh vegetables by blending and drinking the juice without any additive or preservative. Alternatively, get pigweed and prepare gravy with it. It is a laxative that improves your overall health. The gravy with cold rice water can cure dysuria, prickly heat, body heat, coup rap, typhoid, jaundice, herpes chicken pox, and measles.

❖ **Glaucoma**: Drink raw carrot juice and apple juice mixed, and glaucoma will be taken care of.

❖ **Burning urination**: Use black cherry juice. Drink the raw black cherry juice for about 4 weeks consistently and you will notice a remarkable change.

❖ **Bladder and kidney problems**: Drink black cherry juice consistently for about a month and your bladder and kidney problems will go away. Black cherry contains a good amount of magnesium, iron, and silicon, which act effectively as cleanser of the bladder and kidney. Cranberry juice is also a particularly good alternative in the treatment of the above ailment. For bladder problem, you can also use watermelon seed tea. Drink a cup of the tea 4 times daily and early in the evening.

❖ **Peptic ulcer**: Use raw cabbage juice. Note, however that raw cabbage juice causes the formation of gas in the stomach because of its cleaning ability or property. The gas is because of putrefaction in the intestine during digestion. Cabbage juice contains a good amount of vitamin C, A and B. It also has an abundance of mineral elements.

❖ **Arthritis**: Take 2 quarts of carrot juice and 1 quart of celery juice daily for a period of 3 months. This is also good for conditions like neuritis, anemia, and bursitis. Alternatively, get sida acuta plant, make a decoction of it and drink 40 ml of it, 2 times daily for 2 weeks. In case of nervous disorder (Acute), get the root of sida acuta, scrape it with a knife, and dry it. When it is dried, make smooth powder out of it and add a teaspoonful in a glass of boiling water and then take a glassful daily, for 3 days.

❖ **Chronic prostrate ailment**: Use Bee Pollen tablets, 2 tablets, three times a day with food and two (2) just before going to bed, together with 30 milligrams of zinc daily, making 10 mg, 3 times a day. Pumpkin seed is also a good remedy, since it is rich in unsaturated fatty acids.

❖ **Anemia**: Use blackstrap molasses. It is extraordinarily rich in iron and many other vitamins and minerals.

❖ **Itching and cracked skin (skin rashes):** Use 2 tablespoons of blackstrap molasses orally, twice daily for about 4 weeks.

❖ **Shingles:** Get the golden seal herb powder and make a solution of it in boiled water. Then use it to rub the affected area of the skin as needed before bedtime. Also make tea with the same powder and drink it as needed. The golden seal tea is also good for colitis and diarrhea.

❖ **Kidney stone:** Eat banana regularly because according research, banana contains vitamin B-6 (Pyridoxine), potassium and magnesium, which combines with the oxalates in our foods to prevent the formation of kidney stone (calcium oxalate crystal). And drink plenty of water.

❖ **Abnormal menstruation/sexual abnormalities:** Use Wheat germ and Wheat germ oil, 2 spoons 3 times daily. Take the last one 30 minutes before bedtime.

❖ **Heart disease:** Use 2 tablespoons of wheat germ 3 times daily.

❖ **Arthritis:** Alfalfa tea works well for this. Drink 4 cups of alfalfa tea daily, and take alfalfa tablets.

❖ **Cold and sinus:** Use alfalfa tea and 4 tablets of alfalfa every day.

❖ **Typhoid fever:** Get unripe pawpaw (papaya) unripe pineapple, ginger, lime, orange, and Lipton tea. Cut into pieces, and boil with fermented corn water for one hour. Take one glass cup 3 times daily for one week. The ailment will disappear.

❖ **Stomach ulcer**: Get 7 to 8 unripe plantains, peel them, cut them to pieces and pound them; put everything inside a plastic container, fill in with one gallon of water. Allow it to ferment for 3 days. Take one cup 2 times a day for 7 days. The ailment will disappear.

❖ **Rheumatism/Arthritis**: Get 5 seeds of English Pear (Avocado) cut into pieces and dry under the sun and then grind to powder. Mix with a glass of honey to form paste. Take one spoon of the paste, 3 times daily for 6 days.

❖ **Cholera**: Take 3 teaspoons of salt and one teaspoon of sugar, add half spoon of dry gin (a type of alcohol). Drink all as a single dose. The cholera will stop immediately.

❖ **Pneumonia**: Get a handful of garlic cloves, grind them to extract the juice. Drink a spoon and use the juice to rub the chest region and the back region also. This will stop the Pneumonia. Alternatively, collect some grapefruits and lime, squeeze out the juice in a container or bowl. Blend some cloves of garlic, mix all together, and allow it to ferment. Take a little glass cup twice daily and add honey each time.

❖ **Severe cough**: Get about 10 pieces of bitter kola,

grind to powder, add half cup of original honey. Take 2 spoons, 3 times a day for 4 days.

❖ **Stomach ulcer**: Use cabbage. Drink 6 glasses of raw cabbage juice every day for 3 weeks. You will experience a dramatic positive change. Cabbage juice is high in Vitamin C, A, and B. It is also loaded with all the minerals, which contributes to its high value for combating any medical condition.

❖ **Tuberculosis**: Get 20-25 pieces of bitter kola, ginger of equal quantity and 3 bulbs of garlic, blend everything together and add a bottle of original honey. Take one spoon 3 times a day for one month.

❖ **Staphylococcus**: Get 2 pieces of Aloe Vera, cut into pieces, and put it in a container, add one bottle of original honey and a glass of water. Take half cup of it, 2 times a day for one week.

❖ **Pile**: Get the leaves of pawpaw (papaya), scent leaves and bitter leaves, squeeze out the water or juice and mix them together, then take half a cup, 2 times a day for 4 days.

❖ **Woman in difficult labour**: Get some Cochorus Olitorus (Vegetable leaves), squeeze out the water and give it to the woman. The baby will be delivered instantly.

❖ **Menstruation problem in women**: Get 4 to 5 kola nuts, ginger, and garlic, blend them together, and mix with lime juice. Take 2 spoons per day for 3 days.

❖ **Weight loss**: Get some Corn silk, boil them with lime juice. Drink half cup of it per day for one week, and embark on physical exercise.

❖ **Fungal infection**: Mix a native soap or baking soda with ground potash, add lime, and apply the mixture after bath. Alternatively, use scent leave (Basil leaves). Squeeze it into a ball and let the juice of it drip out and apply it to the affected area.

❖ **Gonorrhea**: Get 3 to 4 pieces of kola, ginger, and garlic, cut into pieces, blend them together, and mix with lime. Take 2 spoons per day until it is over. You can also get the root of Aspilia Africana (also known as haemorrhage plant) and crush it with water, then drink a glassful 2 times daily, for 2 weeks. It is also useful in the treatment of sore throat intestinal worms, dysentery, and diarrhea. It is also an antidote for snake venom.

❖ **Internal heat**: Get a quantity of dry pawpaw (Papaya) leaves and cashew leaves, boil with water and drink half a cup daily for one week.

❖ **Insomnia (Inability to sleep)**: Add 3 spoons of honey into a glass cup of milk; take it all at bedtime for one week. You can also get calcium in the form of dolomite. This calcium is good in the treatment of breast pain caused by menstrual cycle. Also, taking a spoonful or two of honey before bedtime, can help you get a good sleep and lose weight.

❖ **Heart failure**: Blend 12 bulbs of onions and 12 bulbs of garlic together; get 3 bottles of honey and mix everything together. Take 2 spoons, 3 times daily for 2 weeks.

❖ **Low sperm count**: Get a large quantity of guava leaves, pound it, add water to it, and filter it. Drink one glass cup 3 times daily for one week. As you drink it, eat carrot and cucumber every day for two weeks.

❖ **Quick ejaculation**: Get 3 bulbs of Okra, slice them, and get the dry seed of okra too and ferment the sliced okra and the seeds with soda water for 2 days. Take half cup per day for one week.

❖ **Weak erection**: Get 6 bulbs of white onions, blend and extract the juice. Mix the juice with honey. Take 2 spoons 3 times daily for one week. In addition, eat a lot of carrots and garlic every day.

❖ **Vaginal discharge**: Get 3 pieces of bitter kola, some ginger, and garlic, blend them and add lime juice to it. Take 2 spoons, twice daily, for one week. For vaginal discharge owing to gonorrhea infection, collect ginger, garlic, lime, and wonderful kola. Get the lime juice and then blend or pound the ginger and garlic and mix all of them together. Let the woman take a little glass cup 2 times per day for 3 weeks. As this is going on, do not forget to mix native soap and lime juice to wash your vagina with warm water, 2 times daily, in the morning and before bedtime.

❖ **Convulsion in children**: Get one onion, small garlic and ginger, blend all together and mix with palm kernel oil. Give the child to drink and use the mixture as cream for the child's body.

❖ **Fire burns**: Rub the affected area with pure honey daily.

❖ **To boost immune system**: Take pineapple. Pineapple juice is an excellent source of vitamin C. It reduces the risk of viral infections.

❖ **Liver detoxification/Colon**: Take pineapple. Pineapple facilitates blood filtration and oxygenation and allows waste substances to be eliminated easily from the body. It also stimulates liver function.

❖ **Urinary tract infection**: Take pineapple juice. Pineapple juice helps to maintain water retention ability and improves proper functioning of the kidneys. It also helps to eliminate urinary tract diseases. Pineapple juice also helps to lubricate woman's vagina during sexual relations or intercourse.

❖ **Inflammation**: Take pineapple. Pineapple contains the enzyme Bromelain. This enzyme has anti-inflammatory properties, which help to relieve arthritis pain and bone disease (Osteoporosis).

❖ **Low sperm count**: Get Bryophyllum leaves in large quantities, and pound them in a mortar to get the juice out. You would need about 1 liter of the juice. Drink this juice in a small glass every day until the one liter is finished. Bryophyllum is also used in the treatment of cough and cold. It can also be used in the treatment of red butt (red disease) in neonate (new born), big belly button in children, ear pain; simply take the leaves, or leaf, place it close to the fire and allow it to soften. Then squeeze the liquid out of it and drink it or apply to the affected area.

❖ **Diabetes (sugar in the blood):** For diabetes or ANY INFECTION, STOMACH PROBLEM OF ANY KIND, POISONING AND MANY MORE, get alfalfa leaves and squeeze them very well and then add a little water to the juice. Drink one cup every day for 3 weeks or as needed. You can also boil the Alfa leaves with *uda* and drink one cup in the morning and one cup at night for infection.

❖ **Cancer:** Use soursop. This fruit is from the graviola tree. It is a natural cancer cell killer. It is grown in the tropical region of the world. You may also make tea from Chromolaena Odorata leaves and drink a glassful three times daily. You can also squeeze and drink it every day.

❖ **For energy:** Get some key lime, blend them in warm spring water or clean water and drink it every morning before meal.

❖ **Rebuilding cartilage, ligaments and strengthening the knee:** Use Oatmeal, Cinnamon, pineapple, orange juice, honey and then blend everything together. Drink the smoothie every morning on empty stomach to improve your knees.

❖ **Clean your kidney and liver**: Get banana, kiwi, lemon juice, parsley, blend them together and drink it every morning, for 3 weeks. It will detoxify the kidney/liver, improve their functions, and prevent kidney stone. It also comes with antioxidant properties.

❖ **Cancer, diabetes, hypertension, arthritis, and cholesterol**: Use bitter leaves, either by cooking in soup, blending and extracting the juice or just chewing the leaves.

❖ **Asthma**: Get bush milk *(tawa tawa)*, or *ewe emile* in Yoruba Language and pound it in a mortar. You can make tea with it or cook it as stew. Take it 4 times a week for about 3 months.

❖ **Kidney cleansing**: Get Garden Egg leaves, wash them thoroughly, boil them for 10 minutes, and allow to cool, filter into a bottle. Take a glass cup of 280 ml twice every day for a period of 2 weeks.

❖ **Air pollution**: Use Ficus retusa Sp. When this plant is planted in the living room, it helps to improve indoor air quality. Orchid plant too can improve the air quality by absorbing carbon-dioxide from the environment and giving back oxygen.

❖ **Lack of focus**: Use Orchid plant to improve focus and to relieve you from stress. Orchids also help to reduce seasonal ailments like coughs, dry skin, and sore throats.

❖ **Piles, urinary disorder, cancer, and heart disease**: Use radish. It can be eaten raw or cooked. Radishes contain small percentage of potassium, folate, riboflavin, niacin, vitamin B-6, vitamin K, calcium, magnesium, zinc, phosphorus, copper, manganese, and sodium.

❖ **Bacterial, viral, and fungal infections**: Use the mangrove plants. They contain compounds that are antifungal, antibacterial, and antiviral. The plants are a rich source of steroids like triterpenes, tannins, alkaloids, saponins and flavonoids.

❖ **Swelling, ulcer and nervous affliction of children**: Use the roots of spider lily. Decoction of it is used to neutralize poison. Boil it in water. Drink it as needed.

❖ **Joint aches**: Use Rose Balsam. Cook the leaves and young shoots. The seed can be eaten raw or cooked, but the seeds are difficult to collect because of the explosive mechanism nature of the seed. But the plant can be dangerous, due to high mineral content like calcium Oxalate, which can cause kidney stone. But when cooked thoroughly, the calcium Oxalate is destroyed. It can also be thoroughly dried to get rid of the Calcium Oxalate.

❖ **Constipation**: Use Morning Glory, by brewing it as tea to make a very potent laxative. The flower also can be made into laxative to purge the system. But be careful not to consume the morning glory seeds, as this can cause hallucination.

❖ **Erectile dysfunction:**

- Get watermelon, Turmeric, ginger, and garlic onion; prepare it by blending both the watermelon rind and flesh, and mix with a little bit of blended ginger, turmeric and garlic and then filter it into a bottle. Drink 1 cup, 2 times daily.

- Get one bulb of onions, 4 cloves of garlic, one tablespoon of olive oil and a cup of water. Blend or chop these ingredients, and boil in water for about 30 minutes. You can add honey as needed. Drink this every morning before breakfast and at night before dinner.

For stronger erection, eat the following:

- Oysters with Shell: Rich in zinc to boost testosterone, enhance libido, and develop sex organs.

- Dark chocolate: Raw and unsweetened is good for aphrodisiac purpose.

- Garlic: For testosterone boosting and libido. It makes the blood flow freely to the genital area.

- Onions: Enhances longer and stronger erection by increasing the blood volume and maintaining a good heart health.

- Saffron: Makes the body sensitive to touch and feelings, thus increasing libido. Take it with milk at or before bedtime.

- Citrus fruits: High in Vitamin C; it increases nitric oxide that relaxes the arteries and reduces blood pressure for better circulation, leading to good erection.

- Chilies: This contains alkaloids, which improve circulation. It also boosts nitric oxide, reduces blood pressure, and makes the blood flow to the genital area.

- Watermelon: It enhances the pumping action of the blood to the penis to improve erection.

- Pomegranate: This should be eaten every day, as it will make the penis grow stronger and healthier.

- Banana: This contains potassium and improves blood circulation.

- Ginger; Onions; garlic and cucumber. Blend these 4 items together and drink the juice every day for erection enhancement

- Aloe vera gel, 2 eggs, orange juice, soymilk, almond milk, molasses, 2 tablespoons of flaxseed/linseeds. First break the eggs and remove the eye of the eggs and then pour it into a blender. Add 2 tablespoons of molasses, then add 5 spoons of blended flaxseeds, and 1 cup of orange juice. Cut a piece of Aloe-Vera gel into the blender cup, and then blend it to smoothie. Drink it every morning before breakfast and before bedtime.

❖ **Pyonephrosis (kidney disorder)**: Get raw carrot juice, green drink made from celery and cabbage. Drink 1 gallon of carrot juice daily and half gallon of green drink daily.

❖ **Lack of energy**: Get brewer's yeast. Add one tablespoon of brewer's yeast powder in a glass of water, stir properly and drink it two times daily. Brewer's yeast contains 19 amino acids, making it a complete protein; also, it has all the B vitamins, except vitamin A, E, C and 18 minerals. When tired and worn out, go for brewer's yeast.

❖ **Rheumatoid arthritis and rheumatism**: Get alfalfa tea and alfalfa tablets. Drink 5 cups of alfalfa tea and 35 alfalfa tablets every day for a period of about 3 to 4 months.

❖ **Heart disease**: Get wheat germ and vitamin E. It is available in capsules and granules. Wheat germ and vitamin E prevent cardiac arrest and restore the heart health.

❖ **Premature aging**: This can be attributed to calcium deficiency. Get about 2,000mg of calcium supplement daily, that is, calcium in the form of dolomite. This can also help in cases of heart palpitation, numbness and tingling in hands and feet (the extremities) and rapid pulse.

❖ **Hot flashes:** This can be due to menopause in women or adrenal rush from dangerous situation on a general note. Get avocado, spinach, kale, almond and turnip greens for vitamin E and calcium. Blend them all together and drink as needed.

❖ **Acne vulgaris:** Pimples on the face. Get ginger, garlic, and rosemary plant. Boil them together and drink as needed. Apply tea tree oil on affected part of the face as needed.

❖ **Aphrodisiac for men:** Get 5 bitter kolas, 5 cloves of garlic, a piece of ginger; blend them together and soak in 1 liter of water. Drink 30 minutes before or after meal. Ensure that you shake vigorously before drinking. Apart from being an aphrodisiac, it is also effective in management and treatment of sickle cell disease, diabetes, high blood pressure and regulates blood sugar. It heals the fontanelle of babies at birth, and even helps with hepatitis B.

❖ **Low libido in men:** Get bitter gourd plant known as *Efirin* in Yoruba language, scent leaves or Basil. Low libido is a result of blocked arteries and veins, which make it impossible for oxygenated blood to circulate round the body. Squeeze these two leaves together in water to extract the juice. Add a good quantity of water and little salt and drink half cup of the extract twice daily. Another way to treat low libido is to get tiger Nut (*Aya*) Coconut, and Dates (*Debi-no*). Soak the tiger nuts overnight to soften it, and then blend it with the rest of the nuts. Sieve it to extract the milk, and drink 24 oz cup full twice daily. Hog plum leaves are good in enhancing libido. Boil it in water and decant it. Drink a glassful, 2 times a day.

❖ **Asthma and bronchitis**: Get Euphorbia and use it to cook native soup; eat this 2 times a day for about 3 to 4 weeks. Euphorbia is also good for the treatment of mucus in nose, throat, throat spasm, vomiting, hay fever and tumors. Carrot juice is good for treating Asthma. Drink a glass every day for a period of one to two months. You can also get some mango seeds, cut it into pieces and keep under the sun to dry. Grind to powder; then put one spoon of powder into a glass cup of water, stir it very well and drink once daily for 3 to 4 weeks.

❖ **Hemorrhage**: Get Aspilia africana plant. This plant is an anti-hemorrhage that can stop bleeding from cut artery. It is also used to stop bleeding of wounds, and sores. It can heal wounds completely and also good for cardiovascular diseases. Squeeze the leaves of this plant and apply to the wound or sores, or drink the juice for internal bleeding. Watermelon root is also good. Pound the roots and boil it for 5 minutes, then drink a cup full three times daily.

❖ **Maintaining the reproductive organ of women**:

Brew the water of the Siam weed leaves and drink it. Do this by using a coffee machine. Instead of coffee, put the squeezed leaves in the machine.

❖ **Teething problem in children**: Get a mixture of lime juice and honey; let it be equal in proportion. Let the child take one teaspoon, twice daily, until the problem is resolved. If however, the child has high temperature, blend some garlic and add to the above mixture.

❖ **Stroke**: For treatment of stroke, collect some avocado seeds, break them into pieces and dry them after which you would grind them into powder form. Add honey to it. Watermelon root can also be used.

❖ **Goiter**: This is a condition caused by lack of iodine. Sea food like seaweed and other edible plants found in the sea can be used to treat it.

❖ **Beri-Beri**: Use alligator pepper (*Mbongo* Spice or hepper pepper) and ginger. Grind them together and take a table spoonful twice daily for 2-3 weeks.

❖ **Fast heartbeat (Palpitation)**: Collect avocado, and mango leaves, and boil them together. Drink 1 teacup, 3 times daily.

❖ **Syphilis**: Look for melon bunch (*Bara*) madumaro root (*utezi* in edo, *utazi* in Ishan, Nigeria) squeeze all the juice and pour into a bottle of dry gin. Allow it to stay for about a day or 2. Take a little glass cup twice daily, for 3 weeks. Alternatively, get some tobacco leaves, garlic, and ginger. Boil the tobacco leaves and ginger together; when it is cool, blend some garlic and add to it; then take 2 cups twice daily, for 3 weeks.

❖ **Fibroid**: Get unripe or premature palm kernel nuts (Elaeis guineesis) crack the nuts and extract the meat inside. Eat about 30 nuts every day for a period of 13 weeks. The fibroid will disappear.

❖ **Bed-wetting**: Get scent leaves, bitter leaves, and squeeze the juice out of them separately, and mix them together with little water. Let the person drink at once with no leftover. Repeat the process every day for one month.

❖ **Wounds**: Get Siam weed (Chromolaena odorata). All you need to do is to squeeze the leaves until the juice comes out, and then spread it on the surface of the wound.

❖ **Headache**: Collect moringa oleifera leaves (the Igbos call it *okwe olu*). Squeeze the leaves to a paste and plaster it on your forehead. This will relieve you of the headache. You can also drink it when water is added to the paste.

❖ **Bleeding after childbirth**: Collect the root of plantain, squeeze out the liquid, and let the woman drink at least 2 to 3 spoonful of it. The bleeding will stop.

❖ **To prevent heart attack**: Get apple cider vinegar, turmeric, black pepper, honey, cayenne pepper and lemon. In 240 ml of water, add 1 spoonful of apple cider vinegar, 1 teaspoon of turmeric and ½ a spoon of black pepper, add 2 teaspoons of honey, or stevia, add one teaspoon of cayenne pepper and lemon juice, then mix the drink very well until everything is well dissolved. This procedure is particularly good to clear the arteries, when the arteries are clogged or to prevent clogging of the arteries.

❖ **To clean up arteries, prevent heart attack and stroke**: Get spinach, turmeric, nuts, like almond and walnuts, olive oil good for cooking, watermelon, chamomile tea, hibiscuses tea, ginger tea, and green tea, and avocado. Exercise is beneficial.

❖ **Typhoid fever treatment**: Get Almond milk, onions, and garlic. Blend the onions and garlic together, and boil in the almond milk for about 15 minutes. When cool, drink half cup or glass on empty stomach. 2 times daily, for about 2 weeks.

❖ **For erection in men**: Get watermelon and lemon. Cut the watermelon, blend, and boil it for about 10 minutes; add the lemon juice to it and continue boiling until the water evaporates and the content in the pot reduces by half. Then, allow it to cool and drink it. Do not take sugar or salt when taking the drink.

❖ **To prevent kidney damage and liver failure**: Get the leaves of the plant, Thaumatococcus daniellii. Boil or steam them and extract the decoction. Drink a glassful 2 times daily for 4 weeks. This leaf is locally known as *moi-moi* (steamed bean pudding) leaf in Nigeria.

❖ **Production of red blood cells**: Get African velvet tamarind. It facilitates red blood cells production, and acts as pain reliever. It also treats dry eye. Eat it straight or dissolve it in water and drink the solution as needed.

❖ **Dengue fever, liver cirrhosis, malaria, cancer, indigestion, and diabetes**: Get the leaves of papaya, blend it, and boil it to make tea out of it. Drink a cup full three times a day, for four weeks.

❖ **Sperm motility and activation**: Get the bryophyllum leaves; pound them in a mortar to get up to 1-liter juice out. Drink a shot once daily, until it is exhausted. Drops of this juice can also cure ear pain. In the case of headache, heat the leaves on fire to soften it and place it on your forehead. Bryophyllum also cures cough, cold, urinogenital infection, red butt in the neonate and the navel of the child.

❖ **For good eyesight**: Drink carrot juice with olive oil. Eat antioxidant rich food. Avoid straining your eyes.

❖ **To boost energy**: Get some key lime and squeeze about 4 to 5 of it into warm clean water and drink it before breakfast and after dinner. This will increase your energy level and ease constipation.

❖ **Treatment of cartilage, knee muscle and ligaments**: Get oatmeal, pineapple, cinnamon, and orange. Blend these items together and drink it before breakfast every day. Only remove the skin of the orange and leave the white pulp under the orange skin, as this will yield better result.

❖ **To maintain good kidneys**: Get kiwi, parsley, banana, and lemon juice. Blend these four items together and drink it every day before breakfast. This will clean up and detoxify your kidneys.

❖ Treatment of anemia, heart disease, boost sperm count, prevent bacteria growth: Get fluted pumpkins (Telfairia occidentalis) also known as *ugu* leaf in Nigeria. Cook the leaves into soup or squeeze the juice out of the leaves and consume it. Either way, it will yield good results. You can also cook the seeds and eat it. But the roots of fluted pumpkins should not be consumed, as it is poisonous and toxic when it gets in contact with the mucosa lining of the stomach.

❖ **Appendicitis**: Get green gram, cook, and eat it thrice daily repeatedly for two weeks. Green gram is also called mung beans. They look like green seeds and are cooked the same way as lentils.

❖ **Stomach pain**: Collect some scent leaves (basil leaves), squeeze the juice out of the leaves and drink this twice daily, for one (1) week.

❖ **Ebola**: Get a good amount of bitter kola and eat at least 4 pieces of it thrice daily, until symptoms disappear.

❖ **Epilepsy**: Another treatment for epilepsy. Get the

leaves of marijuana plant and soak them in a bottle of dry gin or the African traditionally brewed gin called *kai-kai* or *ogogoro* in Nigeria. Drink one shot twice daily.

❖ **Cleansing the blood, lowering blood pressure, high cholesterol level, and high sugar level in the blood:** Get hibiscus flower, garlic, ginger, guinea corn straw (*poporo oka* in Nigeria Yoruba Language). Make a tea out of these items and drink a cup full three times daily, for four weeks. You can add a little sweetener.

❖ Chronic obstructive pulmonary disease (COPD): Get cinnamon, preferably Ceylon cinnamon, and mint leaves, boil them together for about half an hour. Drink a glassful of it every day for about two (2) weeks.

❖ **For inflammation, good brain cells, good digestion, diabetes, cancer prevention, low cholesterol:** Get cactus leaves. Prepare a juice out of the leaves or prepare the leaves with eggs. Drink or eat as needed.

❖ **Seborrhea (skin disorder):** Get Tea tree oil and mix it with coconut oil in the ratio of 2:4. Then rub it on the affected part, as needed. Ratio of 2:4 is 2 equal measures of Tea tree oil and 4 equal measures of coconut oil, using the same size of container.

❖ When there is a disease condition associated with the following; leprosy, strokes due to paralysis, heartbeat, conjunctivitis, epilepsy, edema, kidney stone, heart failure, urinary tract infection, week contraction during labor, get the flower of the Lilly of the valley and distil them either by boiling or by steaming them to rupture the flowers, leaves, and roots, to release the various constituents. Drink a little glassful of this twice daily for 4 weeks. This drink is also good for the treatment of gout, it strengthens memory and restores speech to those with dumb palsy (dumb rabies or paralytic rabies)

❖ For treatment of cancer, kidney disease, gastric ulcer, heart disease, high blood pressure, low back pain, liver disease, diabetes, shoulder pain and general debility of the body, make a juice out of raw sweet potatoes and drink a glass full twice daily, for 4 weeks. You can add a little bit of honey to improve the taste.

❖ For treatment of diseases ranging from hemorrhoid or pile, asthma, toothache, HIV, herpes, hepatitis, cold, chicken pox, influenza, malaria, typhoid fever, body weakness, fungus disease, leprosy, liver disease, blackheads, psoriasis, ulcer, sore-throat, cancer, eye disease, skin infection, wound, high blood pressure, to cardiac problems; get Neem Tree, the leaves, roots, stem, bark, seeds, flowers and the twig. All you need is to boil them in water and drink a glassful of the liquid 2 or 3 times daily.

❖ **Coronavirus (COVID-19)**: Get lemon, lime, ginger, garlic, pineapple peel. Cut open the lime, lemon, garlic, and blend the ginger; then boil everything together with the pineapple peel up to (100 degree centigrade). Drink one (1) cup of the hot liquid every five hours daily and use a portion of the decoction for steam inhalation thrice daily, or as needed, until the virus is destroyed in situ. Eat one (1) bitter kola at intervals of treatment. Steam inhalation is when you pour boiled liquid into a bowl and cover your head over the bowl of steam with a blanket. Then begin to inhale and exhale the steam for about 15 minutes.

You can also get garlic, lemon, ginger, and lime. First squeeze the juice out of the lemon and lime, then blend the ginger, the lemon, and the lime skin together to make a paste. Boil this paste to 100 degree centigrade. Then blend the garlic separately and add it to the boiled paste, each time before drinking it. Drink a cup of this every five (5) hours. Note, each time you drink it, add a portion of the lime and lemon juice hitherto extracted the same way as the garlic. Eat one bitter kola at intervals of treatment. In addition, you can also do steam inhalation only with hot water and eucalyptus oil to clear the nasal passages. Tea made from a combination of Cinchona tree leaves, Lemon grass, and Neem tree (*dogoyaro*), along with Lime, Lemon, ginger, Garlic, Turmeric and Key lime, will also be beneficial in the treatment of corona virus.

❖ To expel cockroaches from the house, get onions and baking soda. Chop the onions, add baking soda to the chopped onion, and place it in strategic places around the house. All the cockroaches will be eradicated.

❖ To expel wall geckos from the house, get salt and garlic. Blend the garlic and mix it with the salt, then place in strategic locations around the house. All the wall geckos will go away.

CONCLUSION

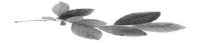

Since man's existence on planet earth (approximately five hundred million years ago, during the quaternary period of the Cenozoic era, only a few seconds before 12 O' clock, according to the geological time scale) man has used herbal medicine to promote good health and longevity. Even to this day, a good majority still use herbs and medicinal plants to meet their health needs. Many orthodox medicines derive their sources from medicinal plants and herbs, save the synthetic medications, which are in most cases hazardous to health.

Today, herbal medicine has gained prominence globally, as its importance has become clear to all, it can hardly be denied by any. Plants and herbs can be used as foods or supplements to meet our daily nutrition needs. For many centuries, certain African, European, Oriental, and occidental countries have been exploring the use of herbs for treatment of diseases and sicknesses. Herbs, in their natural state, have no side effects, as they are in conformity with nature, which is a big advantage over other kinds of medicine. In Africa, the use of medicinal plants and herbs is more prevalent than use of Orthodox medicine. These plants and herbs can be processed and taken in different forms, which includes whole herbs, soups, tea, syrup, essential oils, ointments, salves, rubs, capsules, or tablets that contains powdered form of raw herb or its dried extract.

Over the years, scientists have discovered a decline in effectiveness of some medication for the treatment of certain diseases, which, according to them, is associated with drug resistant traits inherited by disease causing organisms or subsequent offspring of the organisms that have developed some genetic changes by way of mutation. Bacteria, viruses, fungi, etc., are capable of not only changing enzymes targeted by medication, but also utilizing such enzymes to modify the medication itself, thereby making the medication less effective. Therefore, the natural tendency of diseases to develop resistance faster than the rate of development of new medication shows that current techniques for developing potent, long-lasting disease treatment drugs are gradually failing. It is therefore pertinent on the side of government, to encourage the use of natural remedies to counterbalance this failure.

One of the most notable public health risks facing the whole world now is the acquisition of drug resistance traits by pathogenic organisms and the exorbitant cost of these medications. This has necessitated the use of plant medicine. Since there has been no known orthodox cure for coronavirus, at the time of writing this book, the use of medicinal plants and herbs has become inevitable. I am aware of some people who have cured themselves of COVID-19 with the use of herbs like garlic, ginger, lemon, pineapple peel, and so forth. Indeed, true to the words of Hippocrates, the father of medicine, "Nature itself is the best physician."

Made in the USA
Columbia, SC
08 September 2020

18840228R00076